The Biology of Acupuncture

By
George A Ulett, M.D., Ph.D.

Clinical Professor of Psychiatry
Missouri Institute of Mental Health
University of Missouri-Columbia
School of Medicine

and
SongPing Han, B.M., Ph.D.

Clinical Assistant Professor
Missouri Institute of Mental Health
University of Missouri-Columbia
School of Medicine

Warren H Green, Inc.
St. Louis, Missouri, U.S.A.

Published by

Warren H. Green, Inc.
8356 Olive Boulevard
Saint Louis, Missouri, 63132 U.S.A.

ISBN No. 0-87527-534-6

First Printing 2002

This book is dedicated to Professor Ji-Sheng Han whose three decades of careful scientific investigation elucidated the scientific principles underlying this ancient mode of treatment.

CONTENTS

CHAPTER 1
INTRODUCTION

Scientific acupuncture is a simple technique using electrical stimulation of electrically conducting pad electrodes to induce the gene expression of neuropeptides in the central nervous system, thus assisting the body's homestatic healing mechanisms. It is very different from the archaic pseudo-scientific Traditional Chinese Acupuncture (TCA), in which small needles are manipulated in hypothetical meridians to supposedly release imaginary blockages of a mystical energy force called Qi.

This book is designed as a manual to teach physicians this new, user friendly, practical and simple scientific version of an acupuncture-like technique that can be administered within the framework of any clinical practice. It is useful in the treatment of chronic pain and other medical conditions.

Today "alternative medicine" is becoming increasingly popular. There is, however, no alternative to good medical practice. A distinction must be made between those alternative practices that have a sound scientific basis and those that do not. TCA is one of those "alternative" practices that despite its wide use in the United States, is in large part a pseudo-medical placebo. It is typically explained in magical and metaphysical terms and hence shunned by scientifically trained physicians.

When we originally practiced TCA we found it helpful to our patients, but we were uncomfortable with its lack of scientific rationale. It was obvious that acupuncture treatments involved some as yet unexplained neuro-biological mechanism. We had observed surgeons in China adding electrical stimulation to their needles to increase the analgesic effect. In 1972 our laboratory at the University of Missouri obtained the first NIH research grant for the study of acupuncture in the U.S. We found that the addition of electricity to acupuncture needles doubled the relief from experimental pain.

Similar observations had been made earlier by Professor Ji-Sheng Han who had for thirty years been studying mechanisms of pain and acupuncture in his laboratory at Beijing Medical University in China. He demonstrated that it was the electrical stimulation of brain chemistry and not needle placement that was of greatest importance. Conducting pads worked well. With his HANS stimulator he demonstrated the neuro-chemical basis of pain relief by electro-acupuncture. He further established that specific frequencies of electrical stimulation produced the gene expression of specific healing neuro-hormones in the central nervous system (1).

This scientific research was not widely known in the U.S. Here, non-medical acupuncturists have been able to promote legislation requiring extensive training in metaphysics for certification for the practice of ancient traditional Chinese acupuncture. What is being taught is needle acupuncture performed according to the principles of the pseudo-scientific ritual of "meridian therapy". In face of the preponderance of explanatory scientific evidence the ancient practice of traditional Chinese acupuncture is now obsolete. It is kept alive, however, by the media's hunger for exploiting exotic holistic medical techniques and by proponents who sponser teaching seminars to meet state certification requirements established by poorly informed legislators. It is also important to note that as many as 80% of all illnesses are self healing.

How much better to use a simple neuro-physiologically based treatment that adds a demonstrated homeostatic neuro-chemical healing benefit. This manual teaches such a needle-less, neuro-electric stimulation method. This is an effective healing technique that is simple to perform. It can be easily learned by persons with medical training and some basic knowledge of anatomy and nerve pathways. It requires no lengthy memorization of ancient Chinese philosophical beliefs and is compatible with modern medical science. With this text and atlas in hand, any physician can quickly acquire the essentials of neuro-electric acupuncture. Adding this simple technique to their treatment armamentarium will enable physicians to bring to their patients relief from chronic pain and other medical conditions.

Reference:
1.   Han, JS. *The Neurochemical Basis of Pain Relief by Acupuncture.* Hu Bei Scientific and Technical Press, China. 1998. 784 pages.

CHAPTER 2
THE HISTORY OF ACUPUNCTURE

In the Shang dynasty 3,500 years ago, the lives of the agrarian inhabitants of China were dependent upon the changes of the seasons and the vagaries of nature. Hence early religious and philosophical beliefs were tied to a primitive pre-scientific cosmology. As in other world civilizations, healing was by shamans who melded simplistic notions of body functions into a practice combining religion, magic and natural remedies. Concepts of anatomy and body functioning were vague, but early Chinese physicians serendipitously discovered that slivers of bamboo and bone, when inserted through the skin and vigorously manipulated, could somehow bring relief from discomfort in other parts of the body. Thus acupuncture was born.

Huang Di, a fabled Yellow Emperor, was renowned for his interest in medicine and Taoist cosmology. He called together his ministers and a report of their discussions resulted in the *Huang Ti Nei Ching*, *"The Yellow Emperor's Manual of Corporeal Medicine"*, (1). This ancient volume, reputedly written in the Han Dynasty (206 BCE - 220 CE), was copied, revised and interpreted over the years by many authors and has served as a commonly referred to basis for the teaching of Traditional Chinese Medicine including acupuncture.

Confucianism, which became the dominant national philosophy of China, stressed rules for moral and ethical behavior in all aspects of life. It competed with and became a blend with the mystical cosmological interpretations of Taoism. Later this too joined with Buddhism adding yet other mystical beliefs to form the syncretic folk religion of China. These philosophical concepts all played a role in the formation of theories of health and healing.

Dominant in the development of Chinese metaphysics and medicine was a belief in a mysterious body energy Qi. This was thought to course in channels or conduits known as meridians. As in all early cultures, superstition and numerology played a large role. Hence the number of main paired meridians, 12, happened to coincide with the 12 lunar months and 12 animals of the Chinese zodiac. On these meridians were 365 points where Qi came near the surface and subject to therapeutic manipulations. In addition to the 12 major meridians there are two unpaired and also many other supposed collateral energy channels that connect to organs and acupuncture points. As the physician Qi Bo explained to the Yellow Emperor, "The luo collaterals connect with the 365 points and correspond to the 365 days of the year".

The concept of opposites, Yin and Yang, important for a balancing of theorized body energy forces, was deemed necessary for good health. Illness was attributed to blockages of Qi or, as stated in the Nei Ching, "All disorders can be attributed to the blood and Qi not arriving at certain streams and valleys and caves". The latter term being an analogy for acupoints also known as *hsueh*, or hollow spots on the skin where Qi was believed to come to the surface. Traditional Chinese Medicine from ancient times was concerned with balancing Yin and Yang through modification of life-style using the proper combination of herbs, diet, exercise, massage and meditation. Acupuncture involved the treatment of supposed blockages of Qi by the use of various manipulations of acupoints using needles, finger pressure (acupressure) and the burning of wormwood pellets over the skin or on needles (moxibustion). Diagnosis was made, not only by body observation but also by feeling the character of the radial pulse which was believed to represent the state of health of 12 body organs including an imaginary organ called the "triple heater". Six of the organs were represented on each wrist detected by the character of the pulse felt at specific points over the radial artery. (A collection of some diagrammatic representations of these mystical concepts are shown in Appendix B.)

The Chinese were not alone in their concept of a mysterious body energy such as Qi whose manipulation was believed to produce therapeutic results. In India the spirit was known as *atman*, and yogic practices were directed at moving a mysterious energy *prana* upward towards the head through body energy centers called *chakras*. To the Jains the spirit was known as *jiva*. Greeks spoke of the *pneuma*. Other concepts of an etheric body went by different names and descriptions in other cultures.

While the Chinese were concerned with Qi and meridian theory, the West developed the hydraulic theory (Figure 1). This was a belief that pulsations seen in the living brain of animals sent fluid from the ventricular cavities through supposedly hollow nerves into the muscles. Observed movements were taken as evidence of a body energy. In the 1700's Monro demonstrated that nerves were not hollow tubes and with advancing knowledge of galvanic electricity, the stage was set for scientific experiments leading to our present understanding of the nervous system as the true conductor of body energy. It is an anachronism that some adherents of alternative medicine today have reverted to such mystical theories explaining these by controversial concepts of quantum physics. Biomedicine today explains body energy in practical and useful terms of known metabolic processes and the neuro-chemistry of the central nervous system.

Through the centuries in China, the basic doctrine and methodology of acupuncture as described in the *Nei Ching* became greatly elaborated and intertwined with other concepts of cosmology and Chinese medicine. Individual acupuncturists developed their own techniques and added additional special points now approaching the number 1,000. Teaching was by apprenticeship and by the 18th century it was said that it required a lifetime to learn the full body of knowledge required to become a master acupuncturist.

By the year 500 C.E., acupuncture had spread to Korea and Japan and in the 1700's was introduced into Europe by Christian missionaries. Western ideas of scientific medicine were brought to China by these missionaries. Chinese medicine was influenced by these ideas from the West and in 1882 acupuncture was banned by the Emperor as an impediment to scientific medical

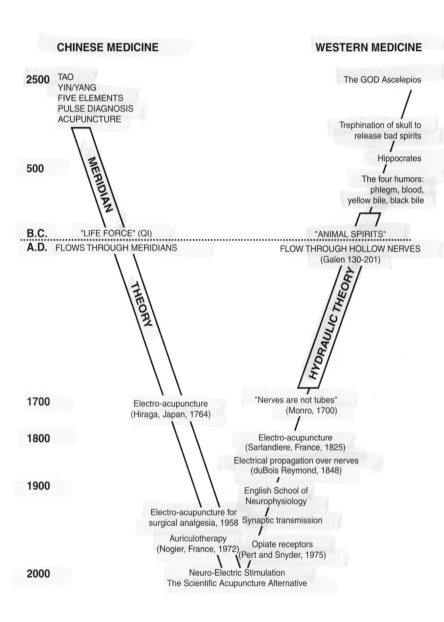

Figure 1.   **Developing Concepts in Neurophysiology and Perpetuation of Myth of Meridian Theory**

progress and it was removed from the curriculum of the Imperial Medical College.

The growth of Western scientific medicine in China was impeded by certain historical events including the Opium Wars and the xenophobic constraints of the Empress Tzu Hsi. Acupuncture was again popularized after the Chinese revolution of 1949. At that time Maoists, faced with a shortage of Western trained physicians and the need to supply some type of medical care to China's millions, instigated the revival of Traditional Chinese Medicine.

An abbreviated method of Traditional Chinese Acupuncture (TCA) was developed and standardized so that it could be taught in an intensive three month course to two million "barefoot doctors". These persons, equipped with *The Barefoot Doctor's Manual* (2) carried acupuncture, first aid and primary care into the countryside. When the "bamboo curtain" parted and President Nixon traveled to China, Scotty Reston, a reporter for the New York Times, experienced relief from post-appendectomy gas pains by traditional acupuncture treatment. Returning to the U.S. he wrote of the wonders he had seen of this "miraculous" method of treatment. The media further extolled the virtues of this exotic "cure all" from the Orient and thus in 1972 was created an insatiable public demand for acupuncture treatments.

American physicians traveled to China and were unimpressed by explanations of Qi, meridians, Yin/Yang and pulse diagnosis. Thus in 1982 the AMA proclaimed acupuncture as "quackery" (3). This was an anathema as far as its acceptance by U.S. physicians. The public, on the other hand, had been thoroughly convinced by media hype that here was a possible miracle cure for ailments that had been unresponsive to conventional allopathic treatments.

Traditional Chinese physicians, previously practicing quietly in isolation in the Chinatowns of America's big cities, suddenly came into prominence. In addition to offering acupuncture treatments they found it lucrative to offer training courses in Chinese acupuncture. Thus in the face of the initial reluctance from U.S. physicians, persons with no medical training entered the practice of medicine as "acupuncturists". Acupuncturists now number an estimated over 20,000 in the U.S.

Traditional Chinese Acupuncture, the method standardized and simplified for the training of barefoot doctors in China, was structured to conform to diagnostic patterns derived from traditional Chinese medicine. Since this was the only established system of acupuncture readily available in textbooks translated into English, it became the U.S. standard. Courses and travelling seminars evolved offering hundreds of hours of acupuncture training. States were faced with the problem of certifying this new brand of practitioner. In the 1980's two national organizations were established to develop standards, the National Council of Schools and Colleges of Acupuncture and Oriental Medicine (NCSCAOM) and the National Commission for the Certification of Acupuncture and Oriental Medicine (NCCAOM). Following their guidelines, states passed legislation to certify the practice of acupuncture. Usually 200 or more hours of training are required.

There has been intense lobbying pressure by persons desirous of "playing doctor" without the necessity of going to medical school. Legislators yielded to this pressure and over 3/4 of the states now certify, under a variety of regulations, acupuncturists who have taken required courses. The requirements vary from state to state. Generally, no medical training is necessary. In some states M.D.'s and D.O.'s can practice with no formal training in acupuncture and in other states non-medical acupuncturists must work under the supervision of physicians or obtain their patients only by medical referral. It is a travesty that in some states M.D.'s whose medical licensure permits surgical procedures are required to take the same courses and pass the same examinations geared for acupuncturists with a high school diploma and no medical training. It has been recently suggested that all persons, including physicians and dentists, be required to have 1,725 hours of training in obscure metaphysics in order to practice acupuncture. Courses vary greatly in content, hours required and cost. Some require three years of training. Fees can amount to $5,000 or more to obtain a course certificate. Ambitious training entrepreneurs have fostered legislation requiring additional hours of yearly updating.

While a few HMO's pay for acupuncture, most third party payers do not, hence lobbying pressure from the national groups persuaded the FDA in 1995 to remove acupuncture needles from "investigational status". This was promoted in order to achieve a basis for Medicare reimbursement for acupuncture treatments. Increasingly, treatments for acupuncture are reimbursable in some states and proposed federal legislation could make such payments universal. The problem is that acupuncture is an umbrella term covering a wide variety of techniques of variable efficacy.

With the introduction of acupuncture into the West, there began a burgeoning of variants from the classical model of traditional Chinese medicine. The now widely practiced TCA is itself a greatly abbreviated version of the classical type of Chinese acupuncture developed over the centuries by ancient practitioners. Korean acupuncture differs from Chinese acupuncture and there are many different kinds of acupuncture in Japan. Some methods depend upon a belief that variations in the measurement of electrical conductivity on hypothetical meridians can produce computerized diagnostic displays and suggest the procedures of treatment to be followed. Ryodoraku, Moratherapy, EAV and Auriculotherapy are hypothesized total systems incorporating different concepts derived from traditional techniques of acupuncture. One of the more widely used methods, Auriculotherapy, has been reported by meta-analysis to be no different from placebo (4, 5). Inasmuch as there is no scientific demonstration of Qi, the possibilities of different varieties of acupuncture treatment are limited only by the imagination. The cult of Qi has also spread beyond acupuncture to become an explanation for other treatments in the field of alternative medicine.

History records that in 1764, Gennai Hiraga of Envo Japan first applied electricity to stimulate acupuncture needles. In 1825, Chevalier Sarlandiere of France used an electric current from Leyden jars to popularize the first electro-acupuncture treatment in Europe. The most dramatic use of electro-acupuncture was reported from China when in 1958 it was used to reduce

dependence upon only chemo-anaesthesia for surgical procedures. Here then was something new. Instead of using mechani-
cal needle manipulation for a supposed effect upon a mysterious
internal body energy, an external energy source was used to
stimulate the body's internal chemistry.

This possibility was intriguing to Professor Ji-Sheng Han,
who observed that the rise and fall of the analgesic effect for
surgery followed the course of electrical stimulation. In his
laboratory, he produced analgesia in a rabbit using electrical
acupuncture. He then produced an analgesic effect in another
animal by simply transferring spinal fluid from the first rabbit
into an unstimulated rabbit. He thus demonstrated that the
analgesic effect was produced by a change in brain chemistry
following electrical stimulation of the acupuncture needle. This
produced an alteration detectable in cerebro-spinal-fluid. This
began three decades of experimentation by Professor Han and
his colleagues at Beijing Medical University that has taken the
concept of acupuncture in an entirely new scientific direction (6).

Pomeranz (7), who co-hosted a conference on the Scientific
Basis of Acupuncture in Nurnberg, Germany in 1987 stated;
"Serious basic research on acupuncture began in 1976 when the
acupuncture endorphin hypothesis was postulated. In the ensu-
ing twelve years (1976-1988) a critical mass of rigorous research
on acupuncture has accumulated". Pomeranz himself contrib-
uted much to this new understanding. His research suggested
that non-responders to acupuncture treatments have a deficiency
in the endorphin pain control system of their brain.

We are now at a time when the cosmology of the ancient
Shang physicians has been replaced by the vastly different scientific concepts of the 21st century. Like the ancient Chinese fable
of the Phoenix bird arising from the ashes, so neuro-electric
acupuncture has developed as a new technique derived from
studies of the obsolescent metaphysics of Traditional Chinese
Acupuncture. With increased knowledge of the involvement of
neuro-hormones in pain mechanisms, Han's new acupuncture
technique has shown that different frequencies of stimulation
can produce the gene expression of different neuropeptides important for the modulation of pain and other central nervous

system activities. It has been demonstrated that this technique is useful not only for pain but also for addiction, psychiatric illnesses and a variety of other medical conditions. Professor Han has developed a method by which electrical stimulation can enhance homeostatic neuro-chemical mechanisms helping the brain to assist natural body healing. He has also demonstrated that needles are no longer necessary. Electrically conducting polymer pads are sufficient. Thus even the terms "acu" and "puncture" are inappropriate. The important work of Cho with fMRI imaging gives added support to Han's findings that neuro-electric stimulation enhances the body's homeostatic regulating mechanisms (8).

It is no longer necessary to spend hundreds of hours learning the magical intricacies of traditional Chinese medicine. Science has made such ancient rituals obsolete. While the path is now open for additional research discoveries, we already have knowledge of what acupuncture is all about. This neuro-electric technique makes available the ability to stimulate homeostatic mechanisms in the CNS for the control of pain and other ailments. Table I summarizes some milestones leading from the ancient cosmology of the Shang dynasty to modern scientific neuro-electric "acupuncture" therapy.

References:

1.   Vieth,I. *The Yellow Emperors Classic of Medicine*, Berkeley, CA. University of California Press, 1949

2.   *Barefoot Doctor's Manual*. The English translation of the official Chinese paramedical manual. Philadelphia, Running Press, 1977.

3.   *American Medical Association Reports of the Council on Scientific Affairs of the American Medical Association 1981*. Chicago: American Medical Association, 1982.

4.   Ter Reit, G., Kleinjen, J. and Knipschild, P. Meta-analysis into the effect of acupuncture on addiction. *Br.J. Gen. Pract.* 40:379-382, 1990.

5   Wells, E., Jackson, R., Diaz, O. et al. Acupuncture as an
     adjunct to methadone treatment services. *Am J Addict*
     4:198-212, 1995.
6   Han, JS. *The Neurochemical Basis of Pain Relief by
     Acupuncture.* Hu Bei Science and Technology Press, China,
     1998.
7   Pomeranz, B. and Stux, G. *Scientific Bases of Acupuncture*
     Springer-Verlag, Berlin, 1988.
8   Cho, Z.H., Wong, E.K, and Fallon, J. *Neuro-Acupuncture*, Q-
     Puncture Inc., Los Angeles, 2001.

TABLE 1
ELECTRO-ACUPUNCTURE HISTORICAL LANDMARKS

1500 B.C.:	Ancient Chinese stimulated points vigorously with slivers of bone
500 B.C.:	TCM - Shamanistic and cosmologic theories of healing
300-100 B.C.:	Diagrammatic lines (meridians connect points)
500 A.D.:	Acupuncture spreads to Korea, Japan and Europe
1764:	Hiraga of Japan uses galvanic electro-acupuncture
1825:	Sarlardiere of France reports on Electro-acupuncture
1912:	William Osler (Johns Hopkins) "advises acupuncture for sciatica"
1958:	China reports on surgery under electro-acupuncture
1965:	Melzac and Wall's "gate theory" of pain control
1972:	President Nixon visits China; Reston reports on "acupuncture cures"
1972:	Wen (Hong Kong) electro-ear stimulation for addiction
1973:	Pert and Snyder demonstrate opiate receptors in CNS
1975:	Kosterlitz and Hughes report on "endorphins"
1977:	Mayer demonstrates significance of naloxone
1977:	Sjolund - electro-acupuncture produces endorphins in CNS
1987:	Han - "Neurochemical Basis of Pain Relief by Acupuncture"
1990:	Han - frequency specific stimulation for various neuropeptides.

Chapter 3
Role of the Placebo Effect

The question has been asked "Is acupuncture a placebo?" The answer is a qualified "yes, and so is every other form of medical treatment." In addition to any scientifically demonstrated neuro-chemical action that mediates treatment there is a placebo component triggered by the factor of belief. In the case of traditional Chinese acupuncture the ambience favors a strong placebo response.

Every family doctor knows the power of the needle. A hypodermic "shot" is better than a pill. Add to this the magic of a media advertised "cure-all" from the mysterious East administered by a magician in a white coat who calls himself a "Doctor of Oriental Medicine". His office has posters marked with strange lines and Chinese hieroglyphics and he performs an impressive ritual with painlessly inserted shiny needles. All the ingredients for a strong suggestive cure!

The word placebo comes from the Greek meaning, "I shall please". Surely, when the treatment is successful both patient and doctor are pleased. For the patient, placebo means "I believe", for when the patient has faith in the doctor and the treatment, the placebo response is strengthened. The physician's strong belief that the treatment will be effective is communicated to the patient verbally and also non-verbally by an air of confidence. And what physician would not feel confident about his beliefs after spending hundreds of hours and hundreds of dollars learning the strange metaphysical rituals of traditional Chinese acupuncture?

But just how strong is the placebo action of acupuncture? Could such a treatment be only a placebo and remain effective for 3,000 years? Traditional Chinese acupuncture has lasted through the ages through its strong placebo action in addition to whatever physiological effect it may have. Throughout the middle ages, medicine in medieval Europe had little to offer except placebo treatment, hope, support and magical rituals. The administration of cupping, purging, plasters and cathartics added but little to the curative effect of placebo, yet civilization survived. Today the public is so accustomed to thinking of medicine in scientific terms that they do not question the deceptive exaggerations of sensational pseudo-scientific media presentation about some of the methods of "Alternative Medicine" (1). Acupuncture is now a household word that is commonly associated with belief in miraculous curative powers.

Although it is usually estimated that the placebo response occurs in 30% of medical procedures, it has been reported in some cases to account for an even greater amount of the treatment result. Most recently even surgery has been shown that it has a placebo action. J.B. Mosley of Texas (2) reported a double blind experiment in which a simple sutured incision on the skin of the knee produced as much pain relief as a genuine arthroscopic procedure. Forty years earlier, Cobb (3) demonstrated that the then popular procedure of mammary artery transplant for angina pectoris was no more effective than a simple skin incision when the patient underwent the impressive ritual of a false surgical procedure.

Today thousands of acupuncturists in the U.S. are overly dependent on placebo action and fail to recognize that there is now available a much more effective technique that surpasses ancient metaphysical rituals. Scientific neuro-electric acupuncture may still carry an aura of placebo but the stronger central nervous system homeostatic action adds greatly to the clinical results.

In 1997, the technique of traditional Chinese needle acupuncture was given significant support following an NIH/OAM Consensus Meeting (4). Clinical presentations to the committee were based on needling of acupuncture points performed in keeping with pre-scientific five element and meridian theories which the report stated, "continue to play an important role in the evaluation of patients and the formulation of treatments in acupuncture". The committee noted that the FDA had removed needles from the category of "experimental medical devices." The committee gave a strong recommendation for the effectiveness of traditional Chinese acupuncture for "adult post-operative and chemotherapy nausea and vomiting, and post operative dental pain and for situations such as addiction, stroke rehabilitation, headache, menstrual cramps, tennis elbow, fibromyalgia pain, osteoarthritis, low back pain and asthma." They stressed the need for implementing better controlled double blind studies. They also noted that "the so-called 'non-specific' effects (i.e. placebo) account for a substantial proportion of its effectiveness, and thus should not be casually discounted."

In 1984 the AMA labeled acupuncture as "quackery" (5), for even then the strong placebo action of acupuncture was apparently recognized. Labeling it as a "quack" procedure, however, effectively discouraged scientific studies of the potential usefulness of this clinical technique by U.S. physicians and medical schools. In the 1970's two leading hypnotists with vast experience in hypnosis (6,7) but little with acupuncture stated that acupuncture was a kind of Oriental hypnotic induction ceremony. As familiarity with acupuncture increased, such opinions changed. Thus Patrick Wall stated in 1972, "My own belief is that acupuncture is an effective use of hypnosis" (8). In 1974, after a study tour of China where he met Dr. Ji-Sheng Han and many other Chinese scientists, he retracted that statement (9). Ronald Katz stated (10) "I have assisted at four operations under acupuncture anesthesia and many more than that under hypnosis. The patients behave differently. Those under hypnosis are seemingly unaware of what is going on around them. Patients under acupuncture were part of the team, joking, laughing and commenting freely."

When President Nixon visited China in 1972, Scotty Reston, a reporter for the *New York Times*, had an appendectomy done under traditional gas anesthesia following which his post-operative intestinal discomfort was treated successfully with needle acupuncture at a point on his leg known as *tsu san li*. As one wag said, "Gas was passed and history was made". Reston reported in the American press the widespread use of acupuncture in traditional Chinese medicine. His personal experience was often misquoted as "surgery done under acupuncture". It is true that in the 1950's Chinese surgeons had reported strengthening the known analgesic effect of acupuncture for surgical operations by applying electrical stimulation to the needles. But the famous cardiac surgeon Michael DeBakey reported in *Reader's Digest*, September 1973, that when surgery was done the anesthesiologists also used such sedatives as phenobarbital and morphine. The patients were carefully selected and only certain types of operations were done. As I witnessed such procedures at a hospital in Shanghai in the 1980's, it recalled my own standard type inguinal hernia repair done under autohypnosis with only procainization of the skin. When I stepped from the operating table and walked to my room, a nurse at the desk queried, "Why Dr. Ulett, I thought you were having surgery today?"

In 1972, our group at the University of Missouri received the first NIH grant to study acupuncture and hypnosis. We used experimental pain and compared the effectiveness of needle acupuncture, electro-acupuncture, intra-muscular injections of morphine and hypnosis for the alleviation of pain (11). We found that electro-acupuncture was equally as effective as morphine and that hypnosis and electro-acupuncture could both effectively modulate the experimental pain. There was, however, a difference between the patient groups. Those who were poor hypnotic subjects did well with electro-acupuncture. Our major finding was that the addition of electricity to the needles produced a 100% increase in pain control (see Figure 2).

Wu et al. (12), using the functional magnetic resonance imaging technique (fMRI), showed that it required vigorous manipulation of the treating needle to effect the stimulation of muscle afferent impulses to produce what is known in traditional acupuncture as the *De Qi* effect. So one can conclude that the placebo magic of the needle can be significantly increased by a stronger type of stimulation. This can also be achieved by using a larger number of needles for a single treatment (13). The addition of a scientific procedure such as neuro-electrical stimulation, given with the proper treatment parameters at only 4

PAIN

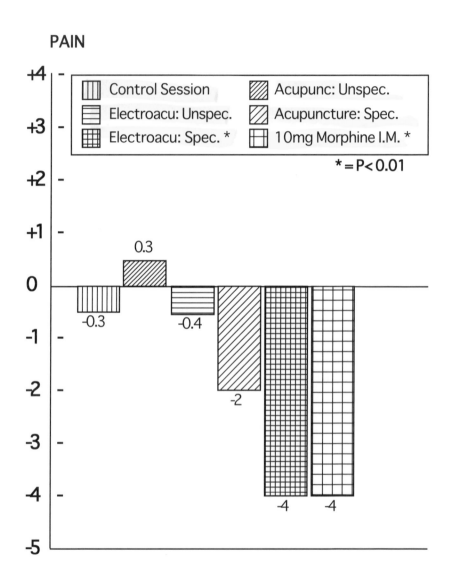

Figure 2   **Changes in Subjective Experience with Different Pain Challengers to Experimental Pain (N:20)**

points, can produce a significant augmentation of whatever psychological factors may be present.

The ancient lore of traditional Chinese acupuncture describes hypothetical meridians that control Qi from many distant parts of the body. This has fostered the concept that distant points, such as on the foot, may for example affect vision or hearing. This has encouraged the development of treatment by formulae which differ greatly from practitioner to practitioner. In a survey of points used for the treatment of headache for example, we found 20 separate acupuncture points combined in various formulae listed by 33 authors as specific for treating headache (14). In support of Professor Han's studies showing that electro-acupuncture is mainly frequency specific rather than point specific, is recent evidence from fMRI studies on crossmodal spatial attention (15). This indicates a mechanism by which stimulation of points in different parts of the body could give the false appearance of specificity.

So in conclusion, why is neuro-electric acupuncture superior to TCA? Traditional acupuncturists with needles, acupressure and moxibustion , weakly stimulate the skin receptors for pain, touch and temperature. If they insert their needles deeply into muscle tissue and mechanically vibrate the needle thus eliciting De Qi sensation (pain, dullness, etc.), they are stimulating those muscle afferents that relay proprioceptive impulses to the brain. Proprioception is a strong sensory input. Every minute of the day, and even during sleep, we are moving dozens of muscles constantly. Such stimuli release endorphins. This every jogger knows. But very few acupuncturists will constantly twirl each needle for an optimal 30 minutes of stimulation. It is time consuming and fatiguing. For the patient it is uncomfortable. Also the acupuncturist has only two hands for many needles. But unmoving needles send fewer impulses to the brain.

Neuro-electric stimulation, on the other hand, sends a constant stream of signals into the central nervous system. These signals can be alternating and of varying frequencies, strong yet comfortable for the patient. This technique directly stimulates nerve trunks. It activates all electrodes equally for 30 minutes. This is the optimal length of time for gene expression of neuropeptides. As longer periods of stimulation can elicit the expression of anti-nociceptive substances, electronic stimulators can incorporate automatic shut-off times. For all such reasons neuro-electric acupuncture is the best possible method for restoring brain homeostasis producing a physiological action over and above any psychological or placebo effect.

References:

1. Ulett, G. *Alternative Medicine or Magical Healing.* Warren H. Green, St. Louis, 1996, p. 246.
2. Mosley, JB. et al. Arthroscopic treatment of osteoarthritis of the knee. A prospective, randomized, placebo-controlled trial. *Am J Sports Med,* 24:28-34, 2000.
3. Cobb, LA. et al. An evaluation of internal-mammary-artery ligation by a double blind technic. *N Engl J Med,* 260:1115-1118, 1959.
4. *National Institutes of Health Consensus Development Conference Statement: Acupuncture.* Nov 2-5, 1997. Revised Draft 11/05/97. National Institutes of Health.
5. AMA Council on Scientific Affairs. *Reports of the Council on Scientific Affairs of the American Medical Association 1981.* Chicago, American Medical Association, 1982.
6. Spiegel, H. and Spiegel, D. *Trance and Treatment.* New York, Basic Books, 1978.
7. Kroger, W. Hypnotism and Acupuncture. *JAMA,* 220 (7): 1012-13, 1972.
8. Wall, P. An eye on the needle. *New Scientist,* 55:129-131, 1972.
9. Wall, P. Acupuncture revisited. *New Scientist,* 4:31-34, 1974
10. Katz, R., Kao, CY., Spiegel, H. and Katz, O. Acupuncture hypnosis. *Advances in Neurology,* 4:819-825, 1974.
11. Parwatikar, S., Brown, M., Stern, J., Ulett, G., and Sletten, I. Acupuncture, Hypnosis and experimental pain. I. Study with volunteers. *Acup and Electrotherap. Res.,* 3:161-190, 1978.

12. Wu, MT. Central Nervous Pathway for Acupuncture Stimulation: Localization of Processing with functional MR Imaging of the Brain-Preliminary Experience. *Radiology*, 212:133-141, 1999.
13. Dung, HC. *Anatomical Acupuncture*. San Antonio, Antarctic Press, 1997, p. 533
14. Ulett, G. and Johnson, M. Two kinds of Acupuncture. *The Digest of Chiropractic Economics*, 36:25-27, 1993.
15. Macaluso, E., Frith, C. and Driver, J. Modulation of Human Visual Cortex by Crossmodal Spatial Attention. *Science*, 289:1206-08, 2000.

CHAPTER 4
PAIN PATHWAYS AND NEUROPHYSIOLOGY

Although acupuncture is a useful treatment for many different conditions its primary use has been for the control of pain. It acts to induce the neuro-chemical pain control mechanisms of the central nervous system. It is by this means that it initiates the pain modulation function.

Like other body systems, pain control is homeostatic. When a body region is injured, impulses from pain receptors send an alarm signal to the thalamus. Pain may be cutaneous (skin), visceral (body organs), or neuropathic (nerve irritation). Suffering is the emotional component that is influenced by such factors as environmental stress, genetic predisposition, or memories of previous pain experiences. Connections to nerve networks in the cortex supply information about the location of the injury

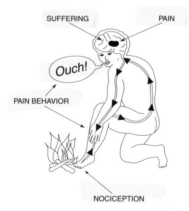

Figure 3.   **The complexity of the pain phenomenon from the noiceptive stimulus to the behavioral response.**

and thus initiate pain behavior (Figure 3). Simultaneously signals from the cortex start the pain modulation cascade through the gene expression of neuropeptides. Activation of nerve pathways originates impulses that descend through the spinal cord.

Nociception, the pain signal, begins with pain receptors in the skin. Here substance P is involved. This pain can also activate the homeostatic mechanism to modulate the pain. This is an essential mechanism to turn off acute noxious impulses for were it not so, we would be overwhelmed by the consequences of each day's bumps and bruises. At the opposite extreme, infants born without a thalamus soon die from accumulating complications of unrecognized noxious bombardment.

The mechanism by which pain initiates pain modulation has evolutionary roots. It produces some comfort for mothers when labor pains induce a rise in endorphin level effecting a lessening of the pangs of pain produced by the tissue stretching that accompanies delivery. This ability of pain to induce some pain relief gives a plausible explanation for the early use of acupuncture. Ancient Chinese doctors apparently found that vigorous manipulation of bone and bamboo slivers could control pain elsewhere in the body.

This lesson has been lost upon many modern acupuncturists whose common procedure is to simply insert extremely fine steel needles according to mystical ritualistic formulae to supposedly relieve the blocking of a mysterious body energy Qi in hypothetical meridians. These needles are often left in place with only occasional twirling. This ritual survives because of its strong placebo effect. Peng and Greenfield (1) have reviewed this matter and have listed some mechanisms that might account for any clinical effects that are observed. Among the factors mentioned are the small current of injury, the reflex release of histamine and the stimulation at nerve endings of the calcitonin-gene related-peptide. The work of Wu (2), using fMRI, has shown that needle acupuncture requires vigorous twirling in order to elicit *De Qi*, an afferent signal from muscle spindles carrying proprioceptive information to the brain. The effects of needle acupuncture are smaller than those of electro-acupuncture but both can be long lasting. Wu's report substantiates the work of Han and others showing that acupuncture stimulation involves basal brain structures and promotes homeostasis. He showed that LI 4 , motor point of the dorsal interosseus muscle, is perhaps the most powerful way to activate anti-nociceptive pathways of the hypothalamus and nucleus accumbens as well as deactivating the rostral part of the cingulate cortex, amygdala and hippocampal structures that play a role in pain perception. Clinical pain control can be evoked by the stimulation of nerve trunks possible with neuro-electric stimulation of either needles or conducting pad electrodes.

From the skin, the pain signal travels over nerve fibers to enter the dorsal horn of the spinal cord. Once signals have entered the dorsal horn of the spinal cord they spread widely throughout the central nervous system. Andersson and co-workers in Göteborg (3,4,5,6), studying pain from tooth pulp stimulation in the cat, ascertained that information interpreted as pain reached the cortex by multiple paths. Some proceeded directly over the thalamo-cortical pathways ultimately terminating in lamina IV of the sensory cortex. Studies from China (7) showed that noxious potentials arriving in the sensory cortex could be abolished by acupuncture stimulation on the hand at the *Hoku* acupoint (LI-4), the motor point of the dorsal interosseus muscle.

The gate theory of Melzack and Wall (8) explained how rapid nerve impulses traveling over myelinated nerves could block the transmission of noxious stimuli travelling slowly over unmyelinated fibers. This would "close the gate" on the upward flow of pain impulses to the brain.

Melzack and Melinkoff (9) raised the pain threshold by stimulating the cat's midbrain reticular formation. Andersson concluded that stimulation of the muscle afferents at intensities activating high-threshold nerves can produce acupuncture effects (10). A sensation of *Teh Chi (De Qi)*, (swelling, drawing, soreness and numbness), that is thought to be essential for obtaining the effectiveness of needle acupuncture arises from A-delta fibers and thus mainly derives from muscle nerves. As noted, injections of novocaine into the skin does not block the acupuncture effect whereas deep injection into muscle tissue can. The widespread nature of pain responses has also been confirmed by observations of an increased cerebral blood flow over large regions of the cerebral cortex after a noxious stimulus (11). This has been clearly illustrated by the animal work of Hand (12), who indexed pain pathways throughout the central nervous system by means of labeled deoxyglucose. He then studied the powerful acupuncture point *tsu san li*, (motor point of the anterior tibialis muscle). He detected a significant decrease in neuronal activity at representative areas throughout the central nervous system pain network when acupuncture was delivered simultaneously with the pain stimulus. Taken together, such explanations clearly demonstrate the electro-physiological component in eliciting the acupuncture effect.

In 1965, Melzack and Wall (8) proposed the gate theory as a mechanism for understanding the modulation of pain (Figure 4). In the years that have followed, an understanding of the mechanism by which pain can be modulated has greatly increased. Han's more complex diagram (Figure 5) clearly delineates anatomic areas and neuro-chemicals that are important in the central nervous system responsible for mediation and control of noxious input (13). Four nuclei; accumbens, amygdala, habenula, and the peri-acqueductal gray, were found to be sensitive

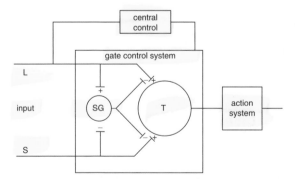

Figure 4.   Schematic diagram of the gate control theory of pain mechanisms. From Melzack, R., and Wall, P.: Pain Mechanizms: A new theory. L=large nerves, S=small nerves, SG=Substantia Geletinosa, T=spinal cord transport. Science, 150:971-73. Copyright 1965, by the American Association for the Advancement of Science.

The Biology of Acupuncture

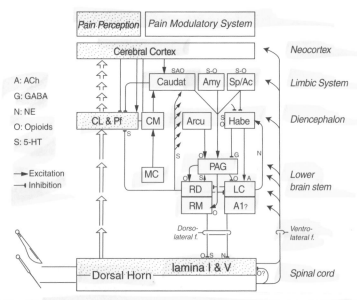

Figure 5.   Diagram showing the possible mechanisms of acupuncture
              analgesia. A1=perikarya of noradrenergic-neurons with de-
              scending fibers to the spinal cord (Whether it is group A1, or
              A5-7 remains to be identified); Ac=nucleus accumbens;
              Amy=nucleus amygdala; Arcu=nucleus arcuatus hypothalami;
              Caudat=nucleus caudatus; CL=nucleus centrolateralis hypo-
              thalami; CM=nucleus centromedianus hypothalami;
              Habe=nucleus habenula; LC=locus ceruleus; MC=nucleus
              megalocellularis; PAG=periaqueductal grey; Pf=nucleus
              parafascicularis; RD=nucleus raphedorsalis; RM=nucleus
              raphe magnus; Sp=septum

areas where naloxone was most effective in blocking acupuncture analgesia. It became clear that there was a mesolimbic loop
(14) with connections between accumbens, habenula, and peri-
acqueductal gray, and that if this loop was broken at any of the
nuclei the impulses necessary for the modulation of pain at the
dorsal horn neurons of the spinal cord would be interrupted.

   It was also found that the hindbrain neural circuits are essential for control of the spinal gating mechanisms. If the upward
flow from acupuncture stimulation is blocked supratentorially
there is considerable interference with the analgesic effect, (14).

The role of the hypothalamus is clearly indicated. Beta-endorphin containing cells of the brain are found in the arcuate nucleus of the hypothalamus and in the pituitary gland (15). From the arcuate nucleus Beta-endorphins are released that stimulate long reaching axons to affect midbrain pain control mechanisms (16). Lesions in the arcuate nucleus can abolish acupuncture analgesia in a rat (17).

Blood levels of beta-endorphin are elevated by stress (18). Although we are concerned here mainly with the effect of acupuncture on pain, it is important to note that other effects of acupuncture (such as upon infections and the immune system) may be attributed to the fact that the precursor molecule, pro-opio-melano-cortin for B-endorphin, is the same precursor molecule from which adreno-cortico-tropin hormone is produced. Thus when an endorphin is produced by electro-acupuncture stimulation, ACTH is simultaneously released.

While such explanations may serve to describe the modulation of acute ongoing pain phenomena, they still leave questions regarding the perception and control of chronic pain. When acupuncture is used as an analgesia for surgery, stimulation is started 20 - 40 minutes prior to the operation. This permits a build up (recruiting, deepening) of sufficient analgesia to allow surgery with a smaller amount of chemo-analgesic. When the electro-acupuncture stimulation is stopped it has been observed that although the effect diminishes, it can last over a period of 30 minutes or more. What then, might be the mechanism for relief from chronic pain over even longer periods of time or as is frequently observed, permanently?

It seems probable on the basis of known physiology that in establishing conditions of chronic pain the ancient, slowly conducting system of C fibers takes dominion over the more phylogenetically recent, rapidly conducting large myelinated fibers. With continuing stimulation from tissue damage or irritation, the pain becomes continuous or chronically intermittent. Such continuous bombardment of the neuraxis by noxious stimuli could well produce a kindling effect (19) within neurone pools of the central nervous system such that reverberating circuits are created with self-perpetuation or continuation of the pain sensation. This type of self-sustaining activity (Figure 6) was described by Lorente de No (20), Dusser de Barenne and McCulloch, (21). Such reverberating circuits at the spinal cord level have been described by Loesser et al in the deafferented spinal cord in a patient with continuing paraplegic pain (22). This self-generated abnormal bursting activity in the spinal cord has also been described by these workers in the cat with chronic deafferentation. Such spinal reverberating circuits could serve to constantly activate pain pathways. This might explain the continuing memory of pain in the central nervous system long after the original tissue injury has been repaired. In the case of phantom

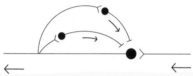

Figure 6.   **Schematic of reverberating neuron circuits in the central nervous system**

limb pain it would appear that the activity continues to reverberate in the central circuits previously utilized by the now nonexistent limb.

An alternative or complimentary mechanism could be a malfunction of the system for production and control of brain neurochemicals that relate to the pain experience. Thus, the noxious impulses could well produce a dysregulation of those homeostatic mechanisms that are normally responsible for a return to the resting stage after the sensation of acute pain has given a warning for the location and severity of tissue damage. A continuing very intense pain stimulus could presumably result in either an excessive production of the peptides responsible for the transmission of pain impulses or a breakdown in the function of those structures responsible for the production of peptides necessary for suppression of neuronal activity in the pain pathways.

Another possible scenario occurs when the pain impulse spreads to involve the intermedio-lateral cell column (Figure 7) of the spinal cord and the sympathetic nervous system neurons located there are activated. Dysregulation here could result in causalgia (23) with burning pain, trophic changes such as glossy skin and often a local rise in temperature. If left untreated, hyper-algesia occurs, muscles become fibrosed, osteoporosis develops and there may occur accompanying emotional symptoms.

Livingston (23) pointed out that, "In many of the causalgic sites which have long been established, the higher centers become affected and all manner of physiologic and even organic changes may take place in parts of the body far removed from

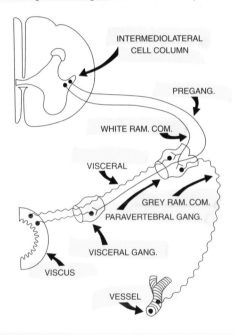

Figure 7.   **Relationship of the sympathetic nervous system to the intermediolateral cell column of the spinal cord**

the original focus of irritation." In some clinical syndromes there may be a combination of somatic, visceral and psychic irritation, each contributing to the central process. Once a vicious cycle is established, the process tends to become self-sustaining.

Other post traumatic pain syndromes as described by Livingston (23), include a peculiar distribution of pain. He speaks of "mirror image" pain in which pain develops in the non-involved side at the precise mirrored location of the contralateral lesion. Such phenomena are explained by the spread of uncontrolled pain by neurons crossing the midline or by spread of excitation by neuro-humors to involve other neuron galaxies in the spinal cord within the same segment but on the opposite side. Livingston has also emphasized the importance of recognizing the neurotome distribution which can be an important principle in acupuncture treatments. An example is his "multifidus triangle syndrome." Here, the innervation of the multifidus muscle by S1-3, may refer pain to both the lateral thigh and the sciatic distribution in the lower leg.

The term "pain memory" has been utilized by Melzack and others to describe long-term chronic pain. The intensity of such chronic pain may gradually abate under the application of repeated electro-acupuncture treatments given over a period of days or weeks. This physiologic effect could thus result from a kindling of activity that inhibits the reverberating pain circuits, or it may be that repeated acupuncture treatments stimulate those neuro-chemical pain control mechanisms that somehow had been lulled into relative inactivity. Acupuncture stimuli thus can bring new life, as it were, into nature's own mechanism for the release of pain-inhibiting neuro-humors.

This brief discussion of neuro-physiology describes some possible pathways involved in nociception. The next chapter describes the central neuro-chemical basis of pain relief by electro-acupuncture.

References:
1. Peng, TC., and Greenfield, W. A Precise Scientific Explanation of Acupuncture Mechanisms: Are We On the Threshold? An Editorial Review. *Acupuncture, the International Scientific Journal,* 1:28-29, 1990.
2. Wu, MT. Central Nervous Pathway for Acupuncture Stimulation: Localization of Processing with Functional MR Imaging of the Brain - Preliminary Experience. *Radiology,* 212:133-141, 1999.

3. Roos, A., Rydenhag, C., Andersson, SA. Activity in cortical
    cells after stimulation of tooth pulp afferent in the cat.
    Extracellular analysis. *Pain*, 16:49-60, 1983.
4   Roos, A., Rydenhag, B., Andersson, SA. Cortical responses
    evoked by tooth pulp stimulation in the cat. *Pain*, 3:247-
    265, 1982.
5. Rydenhag, B., Olausson, B., Andersson, SA. Projection of
    tooth pulp afferents to the thalamus of the cat. I. Focal
    potentials and thalamocortical connections. *Exp Brain Res*,
    64:37-48, 1986.
6. Rydenhag, B., Olausson, B., Shyu, BC., Andersson, S.
    Localized responses in the midsuprasylvian gyrus of the
    cat following stimulation of the central lateral nucleus in
    thalamus. *Exp Brain Res*, 623:11-24, 1986.
7. Research Group of Acupuncture Anesthesia, Peking
    Medical College. The effect of acupuncture on the human
    skin pain threshold. *Chin. Med. J.*, 3:151-57, 1973.
8. Melzack, R., Wall, P. Pain Mechanism; A New Theory.
    Science, 150:971-973, 1965.
9. Melzack, R., Melinkoff, RF. Analgesia produced by brain
    stimulation. Evidence of a prolonged onset period. *Exp
    Neurol*, 43:369-374, 1974.
10. Shyu, BC., Andersson ,SA., Thoren, P. Endorphin mediated
    increase in pain threshold induced by long-lasting exercise
    in rats. *Life Sci*, 8:833-840, 1982.
11. Lassen, NA., Ingvar, DH., Skinh, JE. Brain function and
    blood flow. *Sci Am*, 239:62-71, 1978.
12. Hand, PF., Juang. YH., Liu, CN. Use of the 14C-
    deoxyglucose method in acupuncture analgesia studies
    (abstract). *Acupunct Electrother Res*, 10(4):364, 1985.
13. Han, JS., ed. Cheng, T.O. Physiologic and neurochemical
    basis of acupuncture analgesia. *The International Textbook
    of Cardiology*, 1124-1132, Pergamon, New York, 1986
14. Han, JS., Yu, LC., Shi, YS. A mesolimbic loop of analgesia.
    III. A neuronal pathway from nucleus accumbens to
    periaqueductal grey. *Asian Pacific J. Pharmacol*, 1:17-22,
    1986.

15. Bloom, R., Guillermin, R. et al. Neurons containing B-endorphin in rat brain exist separately from those containing enkephalin: immuno-cytochemical studies. *Proc Natl Acad Sci (USA)*, 765:1591-1595, 1978.

16. Watson, SJ., Barchas, JD. Anatomy of the endogenous opioid peptides and related substances. In Beers RF (Ed.): *Mechanisms of Pain and Analgesic Compounds.* New York, Raven Press, 1979, pp. 227-237.

17. Sato, T., Usami, S., Takeshige, C. Role of the arcuate nucleus of the hypothalamus as the descending pain inhibitory system in acupuncture point and non-point produced analgesia (in Japanese, English summary). In Takeshige C (Ed.): *Studies on the Mechanism of Acupuncture Analgesia Based on Animal Experiments.* Tokyo, Showa University Press, 1986, p. 627.

18. Rossier, J., Guillemin, R., Bloom, F. Foot shock-induced stress increases B-endorphin levels in the blood but not brain. *Nature,* 270:618-620, 1977.

19. Gaito, J. The kindling effect. *Physiol Psychol,* 2:45-50, 1965.

20. Lorente de No, R. Analysis of the activity of chains of intermucial neurons. *J Neurophysiol,* 1:207-244, 1938.

21. Dusser de Barenne, JG., McCulloch, WS. Factors for facilitation and extinction in the central nervous system. *J. Neurophysiol,* 2:319-355, 1939.

22. Loeser, JD., Ward, AA., White, LE. Chronic deafferentation of human spinal cord neurons. *Neurosurg,* 29:48-50, 1968.

23. Livingston, WK. *Pain Mechanisms.* New York Macmillan, 1943, p. 253.

CHAPTER 5
NEUROCHEMISTRY OF ELECTRO-ACUPUNCTURE

Systematic studies of the neurochemical mechanisms of acupuncture have been conducted by Dr. Ji-Sheng Han and his associates at Beijing Medical University (1). This outstanding work has not only removed the veil of metaphysics from the over 3,000-year-old Chinese medical treatment, but has vastly advanced knowledge of the brain's circuitry concerned with pain perception and its modulation. Initially, human volunteers in Dr. Han's laboratory were given electro-acupuncture and their pain thresholds were measured over time. The analgesic effect gradually increased, peaked and then gradually declined.

Although the intensity of this effect varied among individuals, it could be elicited from different points on the body and had approximately the same half life. These observations confirmed the analgesic action of acupuncture and caused Han to believe that some chemical substance was responsible for acupuncture analgesia. This conclusion prompted the use of the technique of cross-infusion of cerebrospinal fluid between two rabbits only one of which received electro-acupuncture. Following the electro-acupuncture, the cerebrospinal perfusate of one rabbit was then injected into the cerebral ventricle of the rabbit which did not receive acupuncture. Surprisingly the pain threshold of both rabbits increased, suggesting that the analgesic action of acupuncture is mediated by substances produced or released in the brain. These substances with their analgesic property had been transferred from one animal to the other. Encouraged by the new techniques of neuro-bioassay, Han then embarked upon a series of experiments aimed at discovering which neuro-humors were responsible for this transfer of analgesic properties. Early studies showed that one of the classical neurotransmitters, serotonin, was important for mediating acupuncture analgesia. It was found that the effect of acupuncture analgesia was markedly decreased when the receptor for serotonin in the brain was blocked by cinnaserine, the seratonin antagonist. In contrast, the effect of acupuncture analgesia could be potentiated by the excessive supply of 5-hydroxytryptophan (5-HTP), -the serotonin precursor. Similarly chlorimipramine, a tricyclic compound that selectively facilitated serotonergic transmission, potentiated the effect of acupuncture analgesia.

Han showed that forebrain serotonin is as important as that of the spinal cord serotonin for acupuncture analgesia. However, the central catecholamine, norepinephrin, was found to have an antagonistic effect upon acupuncture in the brain but was essential for the mediation of acupuncture analgesia in the spinal cord. Thus there is good collective evidence that the monoamines, serotonin and norephinephrine play a role in acupuncture analgesia.

The site of the analgesic action of morphine is the brain.

In the 1960's, Tsou and Zhang (2) reported that the site of the analgesic action of morphine is the brain. They injected a minute amount of morphine into the midbrain close to the third ventricle and the aqueduct and found that it could elict a marked analgesic effect, whereas the same amount of morphine produced little analgesic effect when injected into the blood. This study strongly suggested that the brain might have a special mechanism to recognize morphine and make use of it to modulate pain.

Knowledge of nature's own morphine-like substance, the endorphins, opened up a whole new chapter in pain research. There is much evidence to support the role of endorphins in acupuncture analgesia. Mayer (3) studied laboratory-induced tooth pain in humans, producing acupuncture analgesia by manual twirling of needles in LI-4, the first dorsal interosseus motor point of the hand. In a double blind study naloxone blocked this analgesia while saline did not. Microinjection studies of naloxone into the periacqueductual gray or intrathecally over the spinal cord decreased acupuncture analgesia in rats and rabbits (4). Other sites that do not contain endorphins show no such naloxone effects. It was found that opioid peptides could be grouped into the enkephalins, endorphins and dynorphins.

Working with Terenius, Han (5), using the antibody microinjection technique, showed that enkephalins were mediators for acupuncture analgesia in both the brain and spinal cord. In a carefully conducted experiment Han and Xie (6) also showed that dynorphin antiserum blocked acupuncture analgesia in the spinal cord of the rabbit.

Figure 8 illustrates Han's work using antibodies as a tool for analyzing the action of opioid peptides. It was found that dynorphins were effective in the spinal cord but not in the brain. Thus, in summary, it could be seen that acupuncture could release b-endorphin and enkephalins in the brain and dynorphins and enkephalins in the spinal cord.

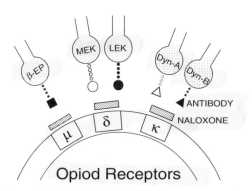

Figure 8.   **Antibody as a specific tool to analyze different kinds of opioid peptides in mediating acupuncture analgesia. b-EP=Beta endorphin, MEK=Methionin-enkephalin, LEK= Leucin-enkephalin, Dyn-A=dynorphin A, Dyn-B=dynorphin B.**

Of signal importance was Han's demonstration in human volunteers (7) that different kinds of neuropeptides can be released in the CNS by simply changing the frequency of electrical stimulation without moving the position of the electrode. Low frequency (2 Hz) electro-acupuncture increases the content of

beta-endorphin and metenkephalin in the CSF, while high frequency (100 Hz) accelerated the release of dynorphin. This
scientific evidence of frequency specific effects that are widespread throughout the CNS is different from the symptom-
specific metaphysical theories of specific acupoint needle stimulation. In 1998 Professor Han published a 784 page review
summarizing all of the studies he and his colleagues had conducted over a 35 year period (1). Essential for consideration by
the clinician, he had not only demonstrated the differential release of brain neuropeptides by different frequencies of stimulation (8) but he also showed that conducting polymer pads were
equally as effective as needles (9).

   Thus from Han's work it was finally possible to describe a
simple clinical method of acupuncture treatment (10) without
the often recommended requirement for hundreds of hours of
lectures on Chinese metaphysics. The following sections review
selected studies that tend to illustrate important areas of Professor Han's lifelong work.*

Acupuncture increased pain threshold in human volunteers with a long latency and half life.

   The first paper demonstrating the analgesic effect of acupuncture using experimentally-induced pain and quantitative
methods to determine acupuncture-induced changes in pain
threshold in medical student volunteers at Beijing Medical University was published in 1973 in the *Chinese Medical Journal* (11).
Pain was induced by modified potassium iontophoresis with
gradually increasing anodal currents (0.1-0.3 mA/step) passing
through the skin on the head, thorax, back, abdomen and leg.
The pain threshold was estimated by the current (mA) needed to
produce pain. Measurements were taken every 10 minutes for
100 minutes after insertion of the needle into the *Hegu* and
Zusanli points, which were manipulated (300 insertion/twistings
per minute, manual acupuncture) for 50 minutes (n=60). Data
was expressed as average percent changes in these skin areas.
Intramuscular injection of morphine (10 mg.) was used as posi-

*This work was supported by the National Institute of Drug Abuse, USA, DA 03983,
and by the National Natural Science Foundation of China, granted to Ji-Sheng Han.

tive control, which produced an 80-90% increase in pain threshold (p<0.05) suggesting that the method is valid. Acupuncture at *Hegu* point produced an increase in pain threshold with a peak increase occurring 20-40 minutes after the needle insertion (Figure 9). The threshold returned to the pre-acupuncture level 45 minutes after the needles were removed, with a half life of 16.2 +/- 1.9 minutes. This result confirmed the analgesic effect of acupuncture. Furthermore, there was no difference in the analgesic effect of acupuncture whether the needle was placed at the left or right hand. Also, a greater increase in pain threshold was produced when both *Hegu* and *Zusanli* points were stimulated simultaneously with acupuncture as compared with the results when either one of these two points was stimulated alone. The analgesic effect was completely prevented by the deep injection of procaine into the *Hegu* point prior to needling.

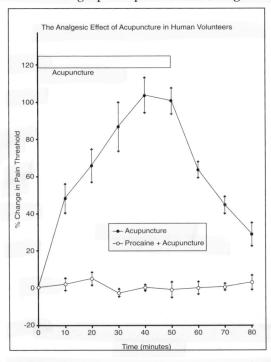

Figure 9.   **Effect of manual acupuncture at hegu point on pain threshold in human volunteers.**

The gradual increase and return in pain threshold suggest that the acupuncture-induced analgesia is mediated by humoral factors. In addition, needling on the affected limbs of 12 hemiplegic and 13 paraplegic patients had no effect on pain threshold on the unaffected side, indicating the involvement of sensory nerves.

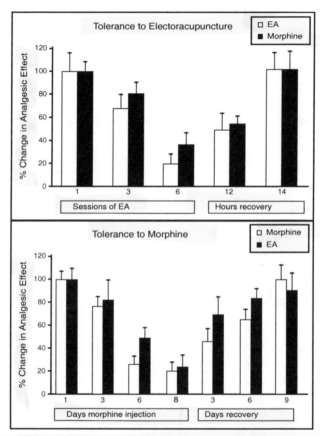

Figure 10.   **Repeated electroacupuncture (EA) resulted in the development of tolerance to EA and the cross-tolerance to morphine.**

Rats developing tolerance to electro-acupuncture analgesia were also tolerant to morphine analgesia.

Several strategies were then employed to characterize the chemical nature of the factors responsible for acupuncture analgesia. Evidence suggesting the importance of endogenous opioid substances in mediating acupuncture analgesia was derived from cross tolerance experiments (12). Repeated electro-acupuncture was applied to rats at *Zusanli* and *Sanyinjiao* points for 6 sessions using 2-15 Hz, 0.3 ms duration, 30 minutes for each session with 30 minute intervals. The amplitude of the pulse was 1 V in the beginning of each session and increased by 1 V every 10 minutes reaching 3 V as maximum.

Repeated electro-acupuncture resulted in tolerance i.e., a gradual decrease of the acupuncture effect (Figure 10). In these rats, the analgesic effect of a challenging dose of morphine (6 mg/kg i.v.) was also reduced correspondingly. The analgesic effect of both electro-acupuncture and morphine returned to the control level at similar rates following a period of recovery (Y=0.78X+22.4, r=0.996, p<0.01). In addition, morphine tolerance developed in rats following chronic injection of morphine (5-50 mg/kg, 3 times/day for 8 days). The effect of morphine returned to the control level 9 days after the cessation of morphine treatment. A similar attenuation of electro-acupuncture analgesia was also observed in these rats (Y=O.74X+28.4, r=0.938, p<0.01). These findings suggest that electro-acupuncture analgesia and morphine analgesia share the same or similar mechanisms.

Acupuncture induced analgesic effect can be transferred to another rabbit when cerebral spinal fluid (CSF) is transferred.

Neurochemical factors responsible for acupuncture analgesia may be produced in and released from the central nervous system. If this is true then infusion of the CSF taken from an animal which has undergone acupuncture into a naive animal might produce a significant increase of the pain threshold in the recipient animal. This hypothesis was tested in a cross perfusion/infusion experiment (11). Finger-acupuncture by pressing *Kuenlun* point (on the top of the Achilles tendon) of the rabbit for

30 minutes produced a dramatic analgesic effect. This was determined by the changes in avoidance response latency during a

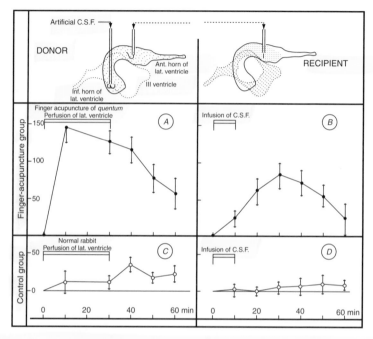

Figure 11.   The analgesic action of acupuncture can be transferred
between rabbits by the transfer of CSF.

noxious stimulation produced by radiant heat from an incandescent lamp (12 V, 50 W in 8.75 mm cine-projector).

The lateral ventricle of the rabbit was perfused with artificial CSF at a rate of 10-15 ml/minute during acupuncture. The CSF from the donor rabbit (0.3-0.5 ml) was then infused into the lateral ventricle of a naive recipient rabbit. A rather marked nociceptive effect was observed in the recipient rabbit (Figure 11). Perfusion or infusion of the ventricle with control artificial CSF had no significant effect on avoidance response latency in donor or recipient rabbits. These results clearly demonstrated that the acupuncture-induced analgesia effect is mediated by substances which are released from the CNS and produce analgesia within the CNS.

Microinjection of opioid receptor antagonist (naloxone) into selected brain regions attenuated the analgesic effect of morphine or acupuncture.

To examine the biochemical and anatomical characteristics of the receptors responsible for acupuncture analgesia, an opioid receptor antagonist was introduced into selected brain regions by the microinjection technique in an attempt to prevent the acupuncture-induced analgesia (13).

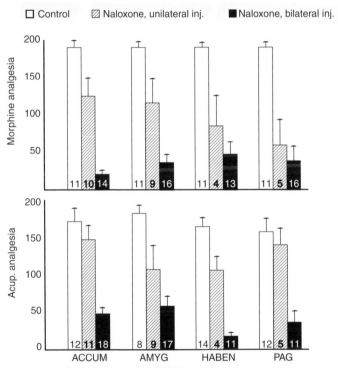

Figure 12. **Microinjection of naloxone into certain brain nuclei attenuates morphine analgesia and acupuncture analgesia. Acup. acupuncture: inj., injection; ACCUM, accumbens; AMYG, amygdala: HABEN, habenula, PAG, periaqueductal gray. Numbers indicate number of subjects tested.**

Intravenous injection of morphine (4 mg/Kg) or finger acupuncture (*Kuenlun* point, 10 minutes) produced a significant analgesic effect in rabbits, as shown by the increase of the avoidance response latency. Naloxone, an opioid receptor antagonist, was microinjected into the following nuclei: accumbens, amygdala, habenula or periaqueductal gray (PAG) at a rate of 0.25 ml/minute for 20 minutes either unilaterally or bilaterally. Microinjection of naloxone into any one of these 4 nuclei significantly attenuated the analgesic effect induced by morphine or acupuncture (Figure 12). These results suggest that the analgesic

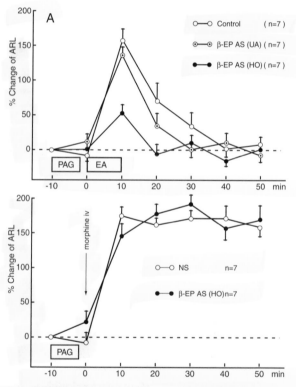

Figure 13.   Microinjection of antiserum against beta-endorphin into the periaqueductal gray attenuates acupuncture analgesia but not morphine analgesia. ß-EP, ß-endorphin; AS, antiserum; NS, normal saline; ARL, avoidance response latency.

effect of morphine and acupuncture is mediated by opioid receptors in these brain areas. Results obtained from experiments using chemical blockade and from studies using lesion methods further suggest that acupuncture analgesia and morphine analgesia may require a neural connection among these nuclei using endorphins as transmitters.

Microinjection of antiserum against β-endorphin into the periaqueductual gray attenuated the analgesic effect of electro-acupuncture but not that of morphine.

At least three kinds of endorphins and their receptors have been found in the CNS. Results from studies using naloxone indicate the involvement of opioid receptors but do not discriminate as to which types of endorphins are involved. Specific antiserum raised against a certain type of endorphin can neutralize and prevent the action of that endorphin. Antiserum which recognizes (HO) or does not recognize (UA) rabbit β-endorphin was injected bilaterally at a volume of 4 μl into the rabbit PAG through chronically implanted cannulae (14). Changes in avoidance response latency (ARL) were determined before and after electro-acupuncture at points *Zusanli* and *Quenlun* for 10 minutes or after the intravenous injection of morphine (Figure 13). The antinociceptive effect of electro-acupuncture, but not of morphine, was attenuated by "HO" antiserum. In contrast, neither saline nor "UA" affected the analgesic effect of electro-acupuncture or morphine. These results suggest that morphine produces an analgesic effect by direct activation of opioid receptors in the PAG whereas the effect of electro-acupuncture is mediated by β-endorphin.

Electro-acupuncture produced corresponding increases in pain threshold and b-endorphin immunoreactivity in the rat brain.

Electro-acupuncture also increases the tissue content of endorphins (15). Rats were divided into three groups according to the degree of analgesia produced by electro-acupuncture (15 Hz, 3V for 30 min.). The electro-acupuncture induced increase in tail flick latency was less than 20%, between 21-70%, and over 70% in groups with low, medium and high analgesic effect, respectively. The brain was removed after electro-acupuncture for measure-

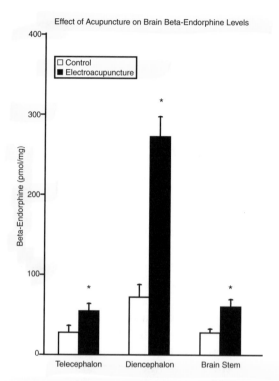

Figure 14.   **Acupuncture produces concomitant increases in pain threshold and beta-endorphin levels (*: p < .05 comparing with
control groups).**

ment of cerebral B-endorphin immunoreactivity (β-endorphin-
ir) with radioimmunoassay. The results show no changes in β-
endorphin-ir in rats with low analgesic effect and a dramatic
increase in β-endorphin-ir in rats with high analgesic effect indicating a strong correlation beween electro-acupuncture induced
analgesia and β-endorphin-ir in brain tissue (Figure 14).

**Enkephalins and dynorphins are selectively released into the cerebral
spinal fluid (CSF) by electro-acupuncture of low and high frequencies,
respectively.**

It would have great clinical advantage if one could selectively stimulate the release of a certain type of endorphin without affecting others. The selectivity of acupuncture on endorphin

release was examined using EA of different frequencies. The spinal subarachnoid space of the rat was perfused with artificial CSF before and after electro-acupuncture at *Zusanli* and *Sanyinjiao* points using 2, 15 or 100 Hz. CSF was collected for measurement of methionin enkephalin, dynorphin A or dynorphin B using radioimmunoassay. Methionin enkephalin and dynorphins were selectively released into the CSF by electro-acupuncture of low and high frequencies respectively (Figure 15). Similar results were also obtained from studies in humans. This conclusion was supported by previous reports showing that a small dose of naloxone, a mu receptor antagonist, selectively prevented the analgesic effect induced by low frequency electro-acupuncture.

Low responders versus high responders for EA analgesia.

It is well known that some people are very sensitive to acupuncture therapy and respond positively after a short period of treatment. A small percentage of people, however, respond poorly to acupuncture treatment. They usually require a longer period of treatment with acupuncture to demonstrate the therapeutic effects. This phenomenon can also be shown in animal studies. When a large group (>100) of rats is given a standard session of EA, one can easily find a bimodal distribution of the analgesic effect. Cluster analysis revealed two distinct groups: one showed an increase of Tail Flick Latency (TFL) no more than 50% (the low responders, LR), the other showed an increase of TFL between 50-150% (high responders, HR). This phenomenon is reproducible at least within several days. What is interesting is that a LR to EA is also a LR to small doses (3-4 mg/kg) of morphine and vice versa. The mechanism of being a LR is at least two fold: a low rate of release of opioid peptides in the CNS and a high rate of release of CCK-8 which possesses a very potent anti-opioid effect. A low responder rat can be changed into a high responder by reducing CCK gene expression with CCK antisense RNA. This can also be achieved by the administration of L-365,260, a CCK-8 receptor antagonist (Figure 16).

The inverse relationship between the responsiveness to acupuncture and the endogenous CCK-8 levels as well as the positive correlation between the responsiveness to acupuncture and

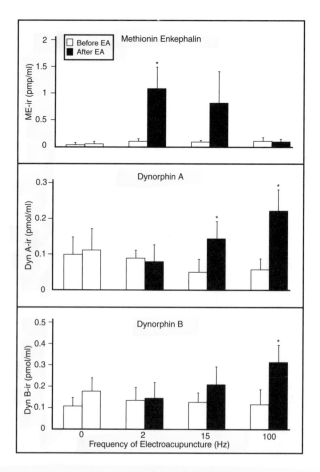

Figure 15.   **Acupuncture of low and high frequencies releases different types of endogenous opiods from the CNS. ME, methionin enkephalin; Dyn, dynorphin**

the central endorphin levels can also be demonstrated in P77PMC rats, which are high responders to EA analgesia. These rats were found to contain high levels of B-endorphin and low levels of CCK in the brain. Furthermore, these animals can be changed into low responders by over expressing CCK gene in the CNS. Thus, a dynamic balance between opioid peptides and anti-opioid peptides in the CNS seems to be a cardinal factor deter-

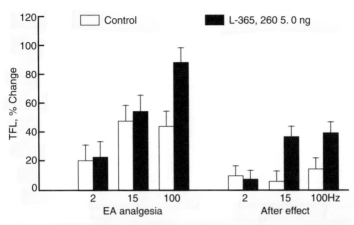

Figure 16.   **The analgesic effect of electroacupuncture was potentiated by intrathecal injection of CCK-B receptor antagonist L-365,260 in rats. EA analgesia is indicated by the average of 3 measurements of tail flick latency during the 30 min. stimulation.**

mining the effectiveness of EA analgesia. It should be noticed, however, that CCK-8 is just one of the many members of the anti-opioid peptide family. Orphanin FQ (OFQ) is the newest member of the family which was discovered recently. OFQ has 17 amino acid residues and seems to serve as a negative feedback control mechanism for opioid analgesia in the brain (17, 18). A decrease in sensitivity (tolerance) to EA may develop during prolonged stimulation. The optimal duration of EA stimulation has been found to be 30 min which is the induction period necessary for the full development of acupuncture analgesia in humans (19). On the other hand, stimulation lasting for more than 1-2 hours would inevitably result in a gradual decrease of the analgesic effect (Figure 17). This can be comparable to the development of morphine tolerance when multiple injections were given repetitively with short intervals, hence the term "acupuncture tolerance" (12).

An interesting finding was that rats made tolerant to 2 Hz EA were still reactive to 100 Hz EA, and rats made tolerant to 100 Hz EA were still reactive to 2 Hz EA (Figure 17). This is understandable since 2 Hz and 100 Hz EA analgesia are mediated by

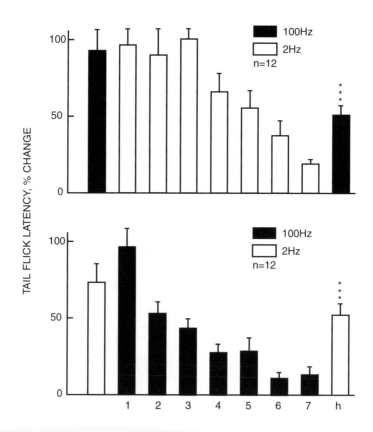

Figure 17.   Rats were given 2 sessions of 30 min EA (100 Hz and 2Hz) to
              assess the efficacy of EA analgesia at these two frequen-
              cies. The 2 Hz EA was then continued for 6 hours. The
              analgesic effect gradually decreased indicating the devel-
              opment of EA tolerance (upper panel). At this point the
              frequency was switched to 100 Hz for 30 minutes, and the
              analgesic effect started to reappear. Similarly, animals made
              tolerant to 100 Hz EA were still reactive to 2 Hz EA (lower
              panel).

different types of opioid receptors i.e., activation of mu opioid
receptors by enkephalin and endorphin in low frequency EA,
and activation of k-opioid receptors by dynorphin in high frequency EA. In the HANS device, a 30 min auto-off mechanism
has been installed to prevent unintentional excessive prolonga-

Tab. I - THE INCREASE OF CCK-8-IR IN THE SPINAL PERFUSATE BY ELECTROACUPUNCTURE STIMULATION OF DIFFERENT FREQUENCIES.

Groups	n	CCK-8-ir (fmol/1.0 ml) in rat spinal perfusate		
		before EA	during EA	after EA
control	8	15.1±1.3 (100)	14.4±1.2 (95)	14.9±1.8 (99)
2 Hz	8	14.5±1.4 (100)	*20.9±2.7 (144)	18.6±1.2 (128)
15 Hz	8	15.6±1.9 (100)	**27.5±3.8 (176)	*22.4±2.4 (144)
100 Hz	8	14.3±2.0 (100)	**25.2±3.4 (176)	*21.9±1.6 (153)

EA was administered for 30 min with increasing intensity of 1-2-3 mA. Data are shown with mean ± S.E.M. of the level of CCK-8-or in the spinal perfusate (fmol/ml). Samples of 1.0 mil in volume were collected every 30 min. n=number of animals in each group. * P<0.05, ** P,0.01 as compared to the corresponding value in the control group.

tion of the stimulation. For severe chronic pain or cancer pain patients who need multiple treatments, it is advisable that the HANS is used no more than 3-4 times (30 min for each session) a day. The mechanisms for the development of EA tolerance are many fold, two of them have been clarified. Repeated EA accelerates the release of opioid peptides which elicits a down regulation of the gene expression of opioid receptors in identified brain areas. The release of a large amount of opioid peptide in the CNS triggers the release of another neuropeptide, namely cholecystokinin octapeptide (CCK-8), to counteract the opioid effect (Table I), (20, 21). Indeed, the development of tolerance to EA can be postponed by the central administration of the CCK receptor antagonist L-365,260, or the antibody against CCK.

Mechanisms underlying the antiopioid effect of CCK-8.

Ample evidence has been obtained to show that CCK-8 forms a negative feedback control for opioid analgesia. It is hypothesized that higher levels of opioids will trigger the gene transcription, protein synthesis and ultimate release of CCK-8 peptide.

This will in turn prevent excessive opioid analgesia. A series of studies were conducted to examine the molecular mechanisms of the interaction between endorphins and CCK-8 (Figure 18). The results of these studies suggest the following mechanisms: (a) There is a cross talk between opioid receptors and CCK receptors. CCK-8 was shown to decrease the number and the affinity of opioid receptors as evidenced by a lower Bmax and a higher Kd in opioid receptor binding assays in the presence of CCK-8. (b) Patch clamp study provided direct evidence to show that opioid suppression of voltage-gated calcium current can be reversed by CCK-8, indicating that opioid/CCK interaction also takes place at the cell membrane of one and the same neuron. (c) CCK-8 seems to induce uncoupling of opioid receptors from their relevant G proteins, thus interfering with the transmembrane signal transduction induced by opioid peptides (22). (d) CCK-8 also antagonizes the action of endorphins by enhancing the phosphoinositide (PI) signaling system in CNS neurons (23) which increases the intracellular free calcium concentration by mobilizing intracellular calcium storage.

In contrast, the opioid effect is to lower intracellular free calcium level. Multiple acupuncture treatments with proper time spacing may result in an accumulation of EA effect. It is known that accumulative therapeutic effects of acupuncture are often observed during chronic treatment. It is interesting that more frequent treatment with acupuncture may not be able to provide a greater therapeutic effect during chronic treatment. For example, the pain relieving effect of long term acupuncture treatments appears to be greater in patients receiving one treatment per week than those receiving seven treatments per week. In normal rats Han compared the analgesic effect induced by EA administered once daily, once every four days and once every week. He found that in the once every four days regime, the EA analgesia showed a trend of gradual strengthening accompanied by a gradual increase of the concentration of monoamines in the spinal perfusate, whereas in the once daily regime, there was a gradual decrease of the analgesic effect i.e., development of tolerance. However, in rats with experimental arthritis, the optimal time spacing for a best therapeutic effect becomes different from that observed in normal rats, depending on the pathological model being used. This is an issue deserving further investigation.

Electro-acupuncture is more effective than manual acupuncture and Transcutaneous Electric Nerve Stimulation (TENS) is as effective as electro-acupuncture.

A series of studies was conducted in rats to compare the analgesic effect induced by three types of stimulation: manual acupuncture, electro-acupuncture and TENS (9). The analgesic

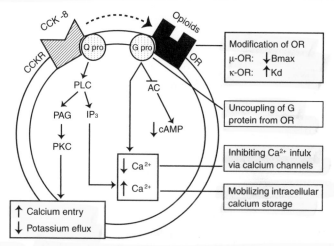

Figure 18.　Diagram showing the possible mechanisms of the anti-opioid effect of CCK-8. See text for details. AC: adenyl cyclase; CCKR: CCK receptor; DAG: diacyl glycerol; G pro. G protein; IP_3: inositol triphosphate; PKC: protein kinase C; PLC: phospholipase C; ↑increase; ↓ decrease.

effect of electro-acupuncture was greater than manual acupuncture, whereas electro-acupuncture and TENS produced similar analgesic effect (Figure 19). Thus the use of needles is unnecessary as conducting polymer pads are sufficient to conduct the stimulus. High degrees of correlation were found between the analgesic effect produced by electro-acupuncture and TENS in individual rats when low (2 Hz, r=0.68, p<0.01), intermediate (15 Hz, r=0.72, p<0.01) or high (100 Hz, r=0.76, p<0.01) frequencies

were used. Furthermore, the analgesic effect of TENS with low
or intermediate frequencies, but not with high frequencies, was
prevented by naloxone. A similar frequency-dependent antagonism was also observed in electro-acupuncture analgesia suggesting that enkephalins and dynorphins are released by TENS
with low and high frequencies, respectively.

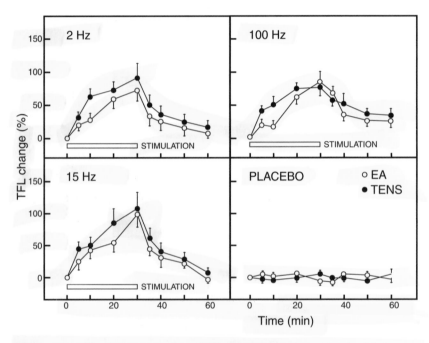

Figure 19.   **Electroacupuncture (EA) and transcutaneous electric nerve
stimulation (TENS) at acupoints produce similar analgesic
effects. TFL, tail flick lantency.**

Optimal conditions for eliciting maximal electro-acupuncture analgesia.

According to thousands of years of experience in acupuncture practice, it is known that different manners of needle manipulation may produce different therapeutic effects. However,
the scientific mechanisms have been unknown. Our study demonstrated that analgesia produced by EA of different frequencies

are mediated by different varieties of opioids in the spinal cord: low frequency (2 Hz) EA analgesia is mediated by metenkephalin via mu and delta receptors, and high frequency (100 Hz) EA analgesia by dynorphin via kappa receptors in the spinal cord (Figure 20).

These results were primarily obtained in rats and recently verified in humans. One could thus anticipate that if low-frequency stimulation appears alternately with high frequency stimulation, both enkephalin and dynorphin will be released successively or simultaneously to produce a more potent analgesic effect via a synergistic interaction between the opioid peptides.

The analgesic effects induced by EA stimulation of various D-D cycles.

Two stainless steel needles were inserted in each hind leg, one in acupoint ST-36 and the other in SP-6. Square waves generated from a Han's Acupoint Nerve Stimulator (HANS) were then measured every 10 minutes. The frequencies for EA were set such that the low frequency was always 2 Hz, whereas the high frequency could be 15 Hz or 100 Hz and designated as 2/15 Hz or 2/100 Hz, respectively. A time cycle of 6 seconds means that low frequency (2 Hz) is alternating with a high frequency (15 Hz or 100 Hz), each lasting for 3 seconds. The

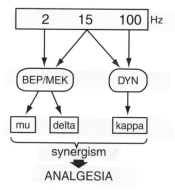

Figure 20.   Electroacupuncture or TENS at different frequencies may release different kinds of opioid peptides in CNS, acting on different types of opioid receptor to produce analgesia.

intensity of EA was increased from 1 to 3 mA over a period of 30 min, at increments of 1 mA every 10 min (Figure 21). The dashed line indicates the average analgesic effect elicited at the three levels of EA stimulation. The results show that the greater analgesic effect was obtained with D-D cycles of 5 or 6 sec., which was significantly higher than that with 2, 4, 8 or 10 sec. per cycle.

Comparison of the analgesic effects induced by EA of 2, 15, 100, 2/15 and 2/100 Hz in rats.

Rats were given 2 Hz, 15 Hz or 2/15 Hz EA stimulation at 1mA for 30 minutes. The TFL was measured before EA and every 10 minutes after the beginning of EA. The mean value of the three post-EA assessments was expressed as percentage change from the baseline level, which was taken as an index of analgesia at 1mA. Similar experiments were performed using 2mA or 3mA instead of 1mA. The analgesic effect of 2/15 Hz was significantly greater than that of either 2 Hz or 15 Hz, respectively. The results from a similar study show that 2/100 Hz stimulation was significantly greater than that of either 2Hz or 100Hz stimulation. No significant difference was found between the analgesic effects induced by EA of 2/15 Hz and 2/100 Hz.

It has been well documented that met-enkephalin interacts not only with delta opioid receptors but also with mu receptors,

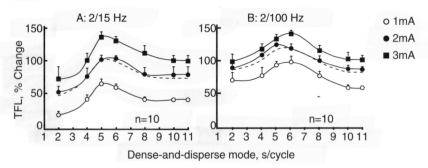

Figure 21.   **The optimal time period for dense-and disperse (D-D) mode of electroacupuncture (EA) stimulation to achieve the best anti-nociceptive effect in rats.**

whereas dynorphin interacts rather specifically with kappa receptors to produce anti-nociceptive effects in the spinal cord. Dr. Han was the first to show that simultaneous activation of two or more types of opioid receptors produce synergistic anti-nociceptive effects (Figure 20). These facts, taken together, may explain the phenomenon that 2/100 Hz EA (which accelerates the release of both enkephalins and dynorphins at the spinal level) produces a more potent anti-nociceptive effect than that produced by fixed-frequency EA stimulation which releases either enkephalins (2 Hz) or dynorphins (100 Hz) in the spinal cord. It should be remembered that the life time of a neuropeptide in the synaptic cleft is relatively short due to the presence of degradation enzymes. The overlapping of the actions of the two neuropeptides will be very brief if the D-D cycle is set for too long such as 12 seconds. In contrast, if the D-D cycle is set at 2 sec. it may not be long enough to induce peptide release to the full extent. These results in animal studies suggest that a D-D cycle of 5-6 sec. is the optimal condition to produce a maximal anti-nociceptive effect. Using a dual-channel constant current electrostimulator (HANS LY257) with two pairs of skin electrodes placed at LI-4 and ST-36 acupoints, similar results were obtained in human volunteers.

From acupuncture analgesia to heroin detoxification.

Since EA has been shown to release opioid peptides in the CNS for pain control, theoretically it should be useful for the treatment of heroin addiction by releasing endogenous opioids to replace the exogenous opiates. This was tested in rats made dependent to morphine (24). The results were encouraging, which led to the clinical observation of using HANS for the treatment of heroin addicts. In the heroin addicts, HANS treatment (30 min. per session, 1-3 sessions per day for 7 days) produced a significant reduction of the withdrawal syndrome. The DD (2/100 Hz) wave was significantly more efficient than the constant low (2 Hz) or constant high (100 Hz) wave in ameliorating tachycardia, insomnia and reducing craving. All three treatment groups using 2, 100 and 2/100 Hz stimulation respectively were equally effective in increasing the body weight as compared to the placebo group in which a gradual decrease of body weight was observed in the first week of drug abstinence (25). After the detoxification period of 7-10 days, HANS can be used for the treatment of various post-detoxification syndromes including insomnia and pain.

An acceleration of the release of endogenous opioid peptides in the CNS may account for the mechanisms underlying HANS detoxification. It should be reminded that 2/100 Hz DD waves releases not only enkephalins and β-endorphin, which work in much the same way as morphine, but also dynorphin which may interact with k-opioid receptors resulting in a suppression of the abstinence syndrome.

Selection of EA parameters should be tailored according to disease category and individual cases

While DD waves have been shown to be the best choice for pain control for most cases, it may not be the standard solution in all cases. This can be seen in the HANS treatment of pain resulting from muscle spasticity caused by spinal injuries (26). Intrathecal injection of dynorphin has been shown to produce analgesic effect in the dorsal horn and may produce paralytic effect in the ventral horn (27, 28). In the condition of spinal spasticity, the anterior horn neurons are in a state of hyperexcitability. It was hypothesized that an increased release of dynorphin in the spinal cord by high frequency (100 Hz) EA might be helpful for a suppression of the excitability of the spinal motor neurons. This was tested in clinical cases of spinal spasticity. Best therapeutic effect was obtained by using HANS of 100 Hz. That of DD mode (2/100 Hz) was only half as effective. 2Hz EA was totally without therapeutic effect and may have even produce a negative effect. The therapeutic effect of 100 Hz EA became increasingly prominent in 5 days and remained stable after 21 days. Another issue worth mentioning is that a low responder rat for 2Hz EA may not be a low responder for 100 Hz EA, and vice versa. Therefore, unless you are sure of the best parameter for the treatment of an identified case, you may try a D-D stimulation first. If it does not work well, then other parameters should be tested.

Conclusion

The studies reviewed here have led to a scientific understanding of the neurochemical mechanisms of neuro-electric acupuncture. This provides the basis for a rational approach for studies of the application of neuro-electric stimulation to clinical problems.

References:

1. Han JS: *The Neurochemical Basis of Pain Relief by Acupuncture. Vol 2*, Hu Bei Science and Technology Press, Beijing, 1998.
2. Tsou K, Zhang CS. Studies on the site of analgesic action of morphine by intracerebral microinjection. *Scientia Sinica* 13:1099-1109, 1964.
3. Mayer DJ, Price DD, Raffi A: Antagonism of acupuncture analgesia in man by the narcotic antagonist naloxone. *Brain Res*, 121:368-373, 1977.
4. Zhou ZF, Du MY, Han JS et al: Effect of intracerebral microinjection of naloxone on acupuncture and morphine-analgesia in the rabbit. *Scientia Sinica*, 24:1166-1178, 1981.
5. Han JS, Xie GX, Zou, ZF, Fokesoon R and Terenius L: Enkephalin and B-endorphin as mediators of electro-acupuncture analgesia in rabbits. An antiserum microinjection study. *Adv. Biochem Psychopharmacol*, 33:369-377, 1982.
6. Han JS, Xie GX: Dynorphin: important mediator for electro-acupuncture analgesia in the spinal cord of rabbit. *Pain*, 18:367-377, 1984.
7. Han, JS, Chen XH, Sun KS, et al: Effect of low-and-high frequency TENS on met-enkepahlin-arg-phe-and dynorphin-A immuno-reactivity in human lumber CSF. *Pain*, 47:295-298, 1991.
8. Han JS and Sun SL: Differential release of enkephalin and dynorphin by low and high frequency electro-acupuncture in the central nervous system. *Acupuncture, the Scientific Internat. J.*, 1:19-27, 1990.

9.   Wang JQ, Mao L and Han JS: Comparison of the antinociceptive effects induced by electroacupuncture and transcutaneous electrical nerve stimulation in the rat. *Intern. J. Neurosci.,* 65:117-29, 1992.

10. Ulett G: *Beyond Yin and Yang: How Acupuncture Really Works.* Warren H. Green Publishers, St. Louis, MO, 1992.

11. Research Group of Acupuncture Anesthesia, Peking Medical College. The effect of acupuncture on the human skin pain threshold. *Chin. Med. J.,* 3:151-57, 1973.

12. Han JS, Li SJ and Tang J: Tolerance to electro-acupuncture and its cross tolerance to morphine. *Neuropharmacology,* 20:593-6, 1981.

13. Zhou ZF, Du MY, Wu WY, Jiang Y and Han JS: Effect of intracerebral microinjection of naloxone on acupuncture- and morphine-analgesia in the rabbit. *Scientia Sinica,* 24:1166-78, 1981.

14. Xie GX, Han JS and Holt V: Electro-acupucnture analgesia blocked by microinjection of anti-beta-endorphin antiserum into periaqueductal gray of the rabbit. *Intern. J. Neurosci,* 18:287-92, 1983.

15. Chen QS, Xie CW, Tang J and Han JS: Effect of electro-acupuncture on the content of immunoreactive beta-endorphin in rats brain regions. *Kexue Tonga,* 28:312-319, 1983.

16. Tang NM, Dong HW, Zhang LX, Wang XM, Cui ZC and Han JS: Antisense CCK RNA and CCK-B receptor antagonist L-365260 changed non-responder rat to responder for electro-acupuncture analgesia. *Chin. J. Pain Med,* 2:103-108, 1996.

17. Tian JH, Xu W, Fang Y, Mogil JS, Grisel JE, Grandy D, and Han JS: Bi-directional modulatory effect of ophanin FQ on morphine-induced analgesia: antagonism in brain and potentiation in spinal cord of the rat. *Brit. J. Pharmacol,* 120:676-680, 1997a.

18. Tian JH, Xu W, Zhang W, Fang Y, Grisel JE, Grandy DK, and Han JS: Involvement of endogenous Orphanin FQ in electro-acupuncture induced analgesia. *Neuro Report* 8:497-500, 1997b.

19. Research Group of Acupuncture Anesthesia, Peking Medical College. The role of some neurotransmitters of brain in finger-acupuncture analgesia. *Scientia Sinica*, 17:112-30, 1974.

20. Zhou Y, Sun YH and Han JS: Increased release of immunoreactive CCK-8 by electroacupuncture and enhancement of electroacupuncture analgesia by CCK-8 antagonist in rat spinal cord. *Neuropeptides*, 24:139-144, 1993.

21. Zhou KY, Sun YH, Zhang ZW and Han JS: Increased release of immunoreactive CCK-8 by morphine and potentiation of mu-opioid analgesia by CCK-8 antagonist L-365260 in rat spinal cord. *Eur J Pharmmacol*, 234:147-154, 1993.

22. Zhang LJ, Wang XJ and Han JS: Modification of opioid receptor and uncoupling of receptors from G protein as possible mechanisms underlying the suppression of opioid binding by CCK-8. *Chin Med Sci*, 8:1-4, 1993.

23. Zhang LJ, Lu XY and Han JS: Influence of CCK-8 on phosphoinositede turnover in neonatal rat brain cells. *Biochem J*. 285:847-850, 1992. 24.

24. Han JS and Zhang, RI: Suppression of morphine abstinence syndrome by body electroacupuncture of different frequencies in rats. *Drug Alcoh Dependence*, 31:169-175, 1993.

25. Han JS, Wu LZ and Cui CL: Heroin addicts treated with transcutaneous electrical nerve stimulation of identified frequencies. *Regulatory Peptides*, 54:115-116, 1994.

26. Han JS, Chen XH, Yuan Y and Yan SC: Transcutaneous electrical nerve stimulation for treatment of spinal spasticity. *Chin Med J*, 107:6-11, 1994.

27. Xue JC, Yu YX and Han JS: Comparative study of the analgesic and paralytic effects induced by intrathecal dynorphin in rats. *Intnl J Neurose*, 82:83-93, 1995.

28. Xue JC, Yu YX and Han JS: Changes in the content of immunoreactive dynrophin in dorsal and ventral spinal cord of the rat in three different conditions. *Intnl J. Neurose,* 82:95-1043, 1995.

CHAPTER 6
CLINICAL USES OF
NEURO-ELECTRIC STIMULATION

Table II lists the many medical conditions which the World Health Organization has found treated by acupuncture in countries around the world. In 1997 the NIH\OCM Consensus Conference on Acupuncture, after reviewing studies using traditional Chinese needle acupuncture recommended the following: There is a potential usefulness and demonstrated "...efficacy of acupuncture for adult postoperative and chemotherapy nausea and vomiting and post operative dental pain and for situations such as addiction, stroke rehabilitation, headache, menstrual cramps, tennis elbow, fibromyalgia pain, osteoarthritis, low back pain, and asthma."

Tab. II - MEDICAL CONDITIONS FOR WHICH ACUPUNCTURE IS COMMONLY USED

Bronchitis and asthma	Conjunctivitis
Coronary heart disease	Acute and chronic rhinitis
Hypertension	Acute tonsillitis
Peptic ulcer	Arthritis
Disease of biliary tract	Shoulder pain
Acute and chronic gastritis	Neck strain
Dysmenorrhea	Tenosynovitis
Morning sickness	Headache
Acute simple appendicitis	Acute and chronic lumbago
Urticaria	Sciatica
Neurasthena	Facial nerve paralysis
Enuresis	Toothache
Intercostal neuralgia and herpes Zoster	Acute sprains
Sequelae of Cerebro-vascular accidents	Vertigo

From: Bannerman, R.H.: The World Health Organization's Viewpoint on Acupuncture. *Amer. J. Acupuncture.* 8:231-236, 1980

These recommendations were based upon the results of studies using traditional needle acupuncture. The use of scientific neuro-electric acupuncture presents even greater treatment possibilities. For, as our studies have shown, the addition of electrical stimulation may even double acupuncture's effectiveness. Thus we have available a simple technique for restoring body homeostasis that could be used to advantage in every physician's office.

Pain

The most common use of acupuncture as reported over the centuries has been for the relief of pain of all types. The usually reported statistic is for relief in about 70% of patients (1). The short lived relief of acute pain may have a higher percentage of success. One of the most widely quoted papers is the exhaustive review of the literature reported by Richardson and Vincent (2). They noted the difficulty in finding a suitable comparable procedure for double blind studies. However, they concluded there is good evidence from the controlled studies reported for the short-term effectiveness of acupuncture in relieving clinical pain. Reported success rates of 50-80% are greater than would be expected if the result were only a placebo effect which is generally in the 30-35% range. Cumulative evidence suggests that acupuncture is a beneficial, cost effective form of treatment for a broad spectrum of acute and chronic pain. It should be made available to patients who fail to respond to other modalities of pain modulation.

In neuro-electric acupuncture treatment the goal is to promote the gene expression of neuro-hormones such as serotonin, enkelphalins and Beta-endorphin that are involved in the central production of analgesia. Thus stimulation of the powerful motor point of the dorsal interosseus muscle is always used for the central control of pain. For pain control at local body areas stimulation of electrodes with neurotome or dorsal root placement can produce release of dynorphins which act at the spinal level. Treatments are given according to the general considerations described herein.

Following these principles, electro-acupuncture with pads and with needles which are sometimes apprpriate, has been successfully used for the treatment of many types of pain. A review of the literature by Birch and Hammerschlag (3) covers a variety of conditions including: facial pain, temporo-mandibular pain, dental pain, neck pain, tennis elbow, osteoarthritis, renal colic, dysmenorrhea, fibromyalgia, athletic injuries, post-operative pain and the discomfort associated with endoscopic procedures. Patients with fibromyalgia report discouraging results from numerous other types of treatment. Combining our usual central endorphin stimulation with neuroelectric stimulation of trigger points, we have had good success with a number of patients suffering from fibromyalgia. The most commonly seen patients in our office are those complaining of headache and low back pain.

Headache

We reviewed 33 articles presenting recommended acupoint formulae for treating headache (4). In Traditional Chinese Medicine, the causes of headache have little resemblance to the usual Western classification of headaches into migraine (vascular) and tension (muscular) types. We found 20 separate acupoints that were recommended in different formulae in the articles as promoted by different authors. We were able to classify the headaches under the general categories of migraine, central, vertex, occipital, frontal and "other". Overall we found that the two most commonly recommended points for treating headache were the Chinese points LI-4 (dorsal interosseus motor point) and GB-20, the point where the tendons of the upper trapezius muscle and the sterno-cleido-mastoid muscle come together in a common tendon attached to the occipital bone. At this latter point there is a liberal supply of Golgi tendon organs. These then are the two points to use for headache. Due to the hairy nature of the GB-20 point treatment using a needle is occasionally necessary. The needle is inserted deeply through the common tendon until the periosteum of the occipital bone is reached. The needle is inserted in the direction of the pupil of the opposite eye.

Vincent (5), reported a controlled series of 14 patients with chronic (mean 3.8 years) history of tension headaches. Patients were given four weekly treatments and followed for 6 weeks with an overall reduction of headache by 59%. Hesse et al (6), reported a series of 77 patients with chronic migraine (mean duration over 20 years). They found that a course of acupuncture treatments can approach the effectiveness of standard medication for the treatment of migraine headaches.

Low Back Pain

Chronic back pain is probably the most common affliction treated by acupuncture. Documentation by clinical reports and controlled studies show an effectiveness of about 70% (7). Thomas and Lundberg (8) compared manual needling and low frequency and high frequency electrical stimulation for the treatment of low back pain. They concluded that only the low frequency electrical stimulation gave lasting results.

In the absence of locating trigger points, the usual treatment for low back pain is to place the electrodes on para-vertebral points (Chinese "bladder points") about one to two inches lateral to the midline of the spine. These are located along the muscle mass in neurotome areas that correspond to the outflow of roots of nerves that make up the distribution of the sciatic nerve. Another frequently used point lies one third of the distance down a line drawn from the greater trochanter of the femur to the sacrum. Increasing the strength of the current may activate motor points of the glutei, obturator internus and pyriformis muscles. Stimulation of other areas along the sciatic distribution can activate motor points of the long head of the biceps femoris, gastrocnemius and flexor hallicus longus. Most commonly used is the motor point of the tibialis anticus muscle (Chinese: *Tsu San Li*, ST-36).

Nausea and vomiting

These complaints may be experienced after general anesthesia, radiation and cancer chemotherapy, during pregnancy and motion (car and sea) sickness. Acupuncture has been tested as a useful alternative and as a complement to standard drug therapy

(9). Most commonly used is stimulation or pressure on the inner side of the wrist on the Chinese point *Neiguan,* P-6. In cases of emesis in pregnant women a combination of points has been used. Stimulation of the dorsal interosseus motor point produces maximum endorphin release and stimulation of the tibialis anticus motor point produces relaxation of the colon. Although some statements in the acupuncture literature warn against the use of lower body points during pregnancy, in our cases it has not disturbed the pregnancy.

Stroke

Researchers from Sweden (10,11) indicate that a program including neuro-electric acupuncture can speed recovery and significantly reduce time in nursing home for patients with stroke. Intervention should be early, within the first ten days. The reported studies used a control group of patients. Both groups received traditional physiotherapy and occupational therapy. The experimental group that showed the marked improvement received, in addition to traditional needle acupuncture, an electrical stimulation at 2-5 Hz for thirty minutes. This was on four needles placed in major muscle groups on the paretic side with stimulation producing muscle movement. Bilateral stimulation with a binaural stimulator on the mastoid areas produced vestibular stimulation.

This study opens the door for further investigation. It is of interest that the investigators were able to achieve improved functioning in severely impaired stroke patients. After one year 25 of the 28 surviving patients that had the neuro-electric stimulation were living at home as compared to only 21 of the 32 control group. The result of decreased utilization of nursing home beds translates into savings in the overall health care budget.

Han (12) showed that in cases of spinal spasticity, thirty minute periods of stimulation with the HANS unit over acupoints on the hand and leg at 100 Hz produced a lasting antispastic effect. Stimulation was conducted daily for three months. He postulated a dynorphin mechanism.

Addiction

Historically, Chinese acupuncturists have long believed that all meridians are connected to the ear and that ear points will control all organs and parts of the body. This theory was expanded by Nogier of Lyon, France (13) and "auriculotherapists" believe that there are 168 specific body and organ controlling points in the ear. Conventional studies of anatomy and physiology offer no support for such belief but recent studies suggest some other possible mechanisms for electrical stimulation of the ear.

In 1972, Wen, a neurosurgeon in Hong Kong (14) reported that electrical stimulation of needles in the concha of the ear was useful in treating the symptoms of heroin withdrawal. This seemed reasonable because the concha of the ear is innervated by the vagus nerve. Electrical stimulation here might produce a broad parasympathetic effect restoring homeostasis and nullifying the strong sympathetic discharge that occurs upon withdrawal from addiction.

In the United States, however, acupuncturists were so convinced of the metaphysics of auriculotherapy that they overlooked the fact that electrical stimulation was essential to Wen's findings. Consequently in the U.S., addictionologists treat by simply placing small unstimulated needles in supposedly specific points in the ear. Meta-analysis of the literature on such treatments by Ter Reit (15) and a recent paper by Wells (16) strongly suggest that this method is mainly placebo. Recently, however, increasing recognition is being given to the fact, in line with Wen's original observation, that electrical stimulation is the essential parameter for any type of acupuncture treatment of addiction.

Katims and colleagues (17) have reviewed the use of afferent nerve stimulation in the treatment of addiction. Included in their review is the work of Ng who used electrical stimulation of the ear to treat withdrawal symptoms in rats addicted to morphine. Han (18), using the HANS stimulator, reported success with acute withdrawal from heroin. Stimulation was at hand and arm points for thirty minutes daily for ten days. He used the dense disperse (D/D) setting which gives three second alternations between 2 Hz and 100 Hz. This treatment permitted acute withdrawal by ameliorating such withdrawal symptoms as tachycardia, chilling sensations, mood changes and weight gain.

Ulett and Nichols (19) report the use of unilateral or bilateral stimulation with electrodes placed over the motor points of the dorsal interosseus and adductor pollicus muscles. Stimulation is for thirty minutes with the HANS stimulator. The method is successful with various drugs of addiction including tobacco, alcohol, heroin and other narcotics, amphetamine and benzodiazepines. In severe cases the HANS is used on a daily basis initially with later spacing as the addiction improves. It is not uncommon to use the stimulus over a period of several months. Treatments may be given with the HANS alone or in combination with methodone and other addiction treatment programs. Some patients learn to use the stimulator at home. In addition to relief from the discomfort of withdrawal symptoms, patients report relaxation and improved mood.

Gastrointestinal problems

Li and coworkers (20) have presented studies showing that stimulation of the tibialis anticus motor point can suppress gastric acid secretion. Chey (21) demonstrated in the 70's with recording of colonic contractions that stimulation of this same point could calm the colonic hyperactivity induced by an injection of cholesystokinin-8. Matsumoto (22) showed during a surgical procedure that stimulation of this point could activate an atonic bowel. I have used this point for patients suffering from nausea and from constipation or diarrhea. At first thought it seems unusual that stimulation of the same point could produce seemingly opposite effects. In the Yin/Yang metaphysics of Traditional Chinese Medicine great emphasis is placed upon the notion that acupuncture balances opposites. As neuro-electric stimulation of motor points can produce the gene expression of important neuro-hormones in the CNS, it is reasonable to presume that such stimulation may promote a homeostatic balance with normalization of body functions. It may also be that with more research we shall find that different frequencies of stimulation can be important in moving homeostatic mechanisms in one direction or another.

Psychosomatic Conditions

There is much emphasis in the New Age literature that physicians in the U.S. should turn to the Orient to learn about a mind/body approach to holistic health care. Somehow it has been overlooked that early in this century these concepts, under the name of psycho/somatic medicine, became important in Western medical training. The concept of homeostasis, introduced by Claude Bernard in 1880 (23), was elaborated by Walter Cannon in 1929 in his book *Bodily Changes in Pain, Hunger, Fear and Rage* (24). Flanders Dunbar in 1945 (25) summarized the 1910-1945 literature on psychosomatic inter-relationships. By that time psychiatrists had demonstrated that the control of anxiety and stress could have a beneficial effect on healing. They spoke of a "holy seven" of psychosomatic disorders including: bronchial asthma, rheumatoid arthritis, ulcerative colitis, essential hypertension, neurodermatitis, thyrotoxicosis and duodenal ulcer.

Today the role of emotions is recognized as important, not in just the above listed seven, but in all illnesses. Contemporary writers like Benson (26) have again emphasized these older homeostatic concepts with new terms such as "remembered wellness". Increased emphasis upon using the patient's own belief system is described in the extensive writings of Larson (27). Studies showing that acupuncture stimulation produces widespread signal decrease in the limbic system suggests its importance for use in treating affective disorders. Thus neuro-electric acupuncture can be helpful in physiologically restoring emotional homeostasis in patients with various psychosomatic illnesses.

To persons familiar with the power of the placebo response, it should be evident that belief is a major factor augmented by the elaborate mystical rituals of shamanic healings and such practices as Ayurvedic and Traditional Chinese Medicine. Patients come to these alternative practitioners with the hope and belief that they will be healed. Traditional acupuncturists are heavily emotionally invested in the belief of what they do. It is also clear that much of what scientific neuro-electric acupuncture-like treatments do is to physiologically enhance the body's ability to mend itself. The demonstrated release of neuro-peptides in the CNS gives assistance to those parts of the central nervous system that are concerned with the establishment and maintenance of homeostasis. Hence the importance of using the HANS stimulator for the treatment of psychosomatic illness.

Wen and Chau (28), reported that electro-acupuncture in the concha of the ear was effective in patients with status asthmaticus. Another point commonly used for asthma and other lung conditions is the Chinese point ST-10 which is located along the anterior border of the sterno-cleido-mastoid muscle near the motor point. Other stimulation may be given over spinal cord roots corresponding to the neurotome of the troubled region. An additional location of stimulation for persons with respiratory conditions, asthma, hay fever and sinus problems is the Chinese point LI-20 in the nasolabial fold. Unstimulated needles are sometimes inserted here at the lower end of the fold and used bilaterally, directed subcutaneously upward toward the nose. This apparently promotes a reflex improvement in the passage of air, hence the Chinese name for this point is *Ying Hsiang*, "welcome fragrance".

These types of treatments are the ones we use for all manner of psychosomatic illnesses. The thumb area is the most significant for the gene expression of healing neuro-hormones. Stimulation of the vagal area of the ear could well be important for balancing the sympathetic and parasympathetic portions of the autonomic nervous system. This logical supposition requires more supportive research.

Depression

A current hypothesis for the etiology of affective disorders indicates a functional impairment of the monoamine system in the CNS. In support of the use of acupuncture for depression, Han has presented data from experimental work on animals. This indicates that electro-acupuncture is capable of accelerating the synthesis and release of serotonin and norepinepherin in the CNS (29). He reported clinical data showing that electro-acupuncture is as effective and has a higher therapeutic index and fewer side effects than amitriptyline (29). Luo and colleagues (30), reported a comparative study treating 307 hospitalized depressed patients with either twice daily electro-acupuncture or amitriptyline for 30 days. The control group of 139 patients received 100-300 mg (average 142 mg) amitriptyline daily. Statistical analysis showed both treatments equally effective but with no side effects in the acupuncture group. This work has been replicated.

As the *HoKu* points appear to be the strongest points, I stimulate these areas when working with depressed patients. Because of third party payer restrictions my experience has been limited to out-patients. I use a conditioning technique that adds relaxation and imagery to the neuro-electric stimulation (31). The results have been favorable and have enabled the use of smaller doses of antidepressant medication.

Conditioned Healing

The knowledge that endorphins can play a role in overcoming the disabling effects of anxiety and stress led us to use the HANS for treating out-patients with phobic and anxiety reaction disorders. We were therefore not surprised when our colleague John Nichols (19) reported from Australia that he had found this stimulation very helpful for some of the Vietnam veterans in his methadone clinic. Once their addiction was brought under control, many were found to be suffering from post-traumatic stress disorder (PTSD). This was considerably helped by continuing the HANS treatments.

PTSD may occur from stress in both military and civilian populations. It is seen in children and adults resulting from single or multiple stressful events. The long term effects of previous stressful events can be compounded or triggered by later happenings and reduce the person's ability to cope. These patients are troubled by recurring, intrusive, distressing recollections of the previous trauma with dreams, hallucinations and dissociative behavior. They may have intense psychological stress with insomnia, irritability, anger outbursts, startle responses, hypervigilance and difficulty concentrating. They typically have complaints of anxiety and depression.

In the course of considering treatment for such psychiatric

conditions, we developed the concept of what we have termed Conditioned Healing with Electro-acupuncture (31). A recent NIH consensus meeting (32) indicated that relaxation is an important part of hypnosis, biofeedback and other treatments for pain and insomnia. Relaxation is an important component of many of the treatments used by practitioners of alternative medicine. Patients usually are relaxed during acupuncture stimulation. It therefore seemed logical to seek to enhance this relaxation response.

Ader and Cohen (33) used Pavlovian techniques to train rats to increase endorphins on a conditioning signal. This suggested the possibility of using such a technique with patients. We decided to use imagery as the conditional stimulus. Imagery has long played a role in medicine with reported ability to stimulate the body's healing mechanisms. Beta endorphins are secreted stochiametrically with ACTH and thus may play an important role in the stress response (34).

Patients are instructed to lie quietly for 30 minutes on a couch while they are receiving electrical stimulation of the dorsal interosseus motor points bilaterally to actuate endorphin release and its gene expression. This is the unconditioned stimulus. Meanwhile they listen to a tape recording that leads them into a state of deep relaxation or self hypnosis. Patients are then asked to recall a relaxing scene from their memory. This is the conditional stimulus. Patients keep such images in mind while neuro-hormones are being released in the brain by the electro-acupuncture conditioning procedure. The patients are then directed to use their relaxing images, the conditional stimuli, while practicing this relaxation technique at home. The goal is to enable the patient to achieve a conditioned gene expression of endorphins in response to a specific personal image which has been used as the conditional stimulus. Because this procedure uses relaxation, hypnosis and imagery in addition to repeated in-office exposure to electro-acupuncture, it is not easy to weigh the individual contribution of each factor. However, patients have universally reported this to be a most helpful combination method for dealing with their symptoms of depression, anxiety, panic states and post-traumatic stress disorder. This is presented as an illustration of how neuro-electric stimulation can be used to strengthen other homeostatic regulation procedures.

Conclusion

It is evident that not only is electrical stimulation essential for the best possible acupuncture-like treatment, but also specific frequencies of stimulus may well be useful for treating different clinical problems. It is not the needles or the meridians and manipulation of Qi that is important but rather the parameters of electrical stimulation that are the salient factors in treatment. As long as the pads are placed in such a way that the electrical stimulation can reach the central nervous system, (i.e. motor points or points adjacent to nervous structures), the archaic rituals of ancient Traditional Chinese Acupuncture are not necessary. What we have now is a simple method, easily learned and quickly applied, for using a specific type of electrical stimulus in order to induce the gene expression of those neuro-hormones deemed necessary for restoring homeostasis.

References:

1. Lu, GD., Needham, J.; *Celestial Lancets*. Cambridge University Press, 1980, p. 427.
2. Richardson, P. and Vincent, C. Acupuncture for the treatment of pain: a review of evaluative research. *Pain*, 24:15-40, 1986.
3. Birch, S. and Hammerschlag, R. *Acupuncture Efficacy: A Compendium of Controlled Clinical Studies*. The National Academy of Acupuncture and Oriental Medicine, Tarrytown, N.Y. 1996.
4. Ulett, G and Johnson, M. Two Kinds of Acupuncture. *The Digest of Chiropractic Economics*, 36:25-27, 1993
5. Vincent, C. The treatment of tension headache by acupuncture: A controlled single case design with time series analysis. *J. Psychosomatic Res.*, 34:553-561, 1990.
6. Hesse, J., Mogelvang, B. and Simonsen, H. Acupuncture versus metoprolol in migraine prophylaxis: a randomized trial of trigger point inactivation. *J. Internal. Med.*, 235:451-456, 1994.

7. Ulett, G. Acupuncture (Chapter 8) in: Tollison, C and Kriegel, M. (Eds). *Interdisciplinary Rehabilitation of Low Back Pain.* Williams and Wilkins, Boston, 1989.

8. Thomas, M. and Lundberg, T. Importance of modes of acupuncture in the treatment of chronic nociceptive low back pain. *Acta Anaesthesiol Scand.,* 38:63-69, 1994

9. Vickers, A. Can acupuncture have specific effects on health? A systematic review of acupuncture antiemesis trials. *J Roy Soc Med.,* 89:303-311, 1996.

10. Johansson, K, Lindgren, I., Widner,H., Wiklund, I. and Johansson, B.: Can sensory stimulation improve the functional outcome in stroke patients? *Neurology,* 43:2189-2192, 1993.

11. Magnusson, M, Johansson, K. and Johansson, B.: Sensory stimulation promotes normalization of postural control after stroke. *Stroke,* 25:1179-1180, 1994.

12. Han, JS, Chen, XH., Yuan, Y. et al. Transcutaneous electrical nerve stimulation for treatment of spinal spasticity. *Chin Med J.,* 107:6-11, 1994

13. Nogier, P. *Treatise on Auriculotherapy.* Maisonneuve, Moulins-les-metz, France, 1972.

14. Wen, H, and Cheung S. Treatment of drug addiction by acupuncture and electrical stimulation. *Asian J Med.,* 9:138-141, 1973.

15. Ter Reit, G, Klijnen, J. and Knipschild, P. Meta analysis of studies into the effect of acupuncture on addiction. *Brit J Gen Prac.,* 40:379-382, 1990.

16. Wells, E., Jackson, R., Diaz, O., Stanton, V., Saxon, A. and Krupski, A.: Acupuncture as an adjunct to methadone treatment services. *Am J Addict.,* 4:1981-214, 1995.

17. Katims, J., Ng, L. and Lowinson, J. Acupuncture and transcutaneous electrical nerve stimulation: afferent nerve stimulation (ANS) in the treatment of addiction. Chapter 8 574-583 in *Substance Abuse: A Comprehensive Textbook.* Lowinson, J. (Ed) Williams and Wilkins, Boston, 1992.

18. Han, JS., Wu, LZ., and Cui, CL. Heroin addicts treated with transcutaneous electrical nerve stimulation of identified frequencies. *Regulatory Peptides*, 54:115-116, 1994.

19. Ulett, G and Nichols, J. *The Endorophin Connection: A Handbook of Opiate Enhancement.* Wild and Wooley, Pty. Ltd. Glebe, Australia, 1996.

20. Li, Y., Tougas, O., Chiverton, S. and Hung, R. The effect of acupuncture on gastrointestinal function and disorders. *Am J. Gastroenterol*, 87:1372-1381, 1992.

21. Chey, W. Personal communication, 1975.

22. Matusmmoto, T. *Acupuncture for Physicians.* C.C. Thomas, Springfield, IL, 1974.

23. Bernard, C. *Lecons de physiologie experimentel applique a la medicine au College de France,* J.E. Bailliere et fils, Paris. France, 1880.

24. Cannon, W. *Bodily Changes in Pain, Hunger, Fear and Rage.* D. Appleton-Century Co. N.Y., 1936,

25. Dunbar, F. *Emotions and Bodily Changes. A Survey of Literature on Psychosomatic Interrelationships,* 1910-1945. Columbia University Press,1946.

26. Benson, H. *Timeless Healing: The Power and Biology of Belief.* Simon and Schuster, N.Y. 1996.

27. Larson, D. and Larson, S. Religious commitment and health: Valuing the relationship. *Second Opinion: Health, Faith and Ethics*, 17:26-40, 1991.

28. Wen, H. and Chau, K. Status asthmaticus treated by acupuncture and electro-stimulation. *Asian J Med*, 9:191-195. 1973.

29. Han, JS. Electroacupuncture, an alternative to antidepressants for treating affective diseases. *Int J Neurosci*, 29:79-92. 1986.

30. Luo, H., Shen, Y., Zou, D. and Jin, Y. A comparative study of the treatment of depression by electro-acupuncture. *Acupunct Sci Int J.*, 1:19-27, 1990.

31. Ulett, G. Conditioned healing with electro-acupuncture. *Alternative Therapies*, 2:56-60, 1996.

32. *National Institutes of Health Treatment Assessment Conference Statement: Integration of Behavioral and Relaxation Approaches into the Treatment of Chronic Pain and Insomnia.* National Institutes of Health. October 16-18, 1996 Bethesda, MD, NIH Consensus Program Information Services, 1996.
33. Ader, R. and Cohen V. Behaviorally conditioned immunosuppression and murine systemic lupus erythematosis. *Science,* 215:1534-1536, 1982.
34. Loh, Y. and Loriaux, I Adrenocorticotropic hormone P-lipo-protein and endorphin related peptides in health and disease. *JAMA,* 247:1033-1034, 1982.

CHAPTER 7
TREATING THE PATIENT

a-Acupoints and Motor Points

By tradition there are some 365 acupuncture points. Over the centuries new acupuncture techniques have added additional points bringing that number to an estimated 1,000. These points are located along hypothetical "meridians" and are thought to be holes, *hsueh*, where the passage of energy, Qi, can be effected to relieve blockages and produce cures. Even among experienced acupuncturists however, the location of acupoints is not an exact science. In our experience, useful treatments can be accomplished by using some of the 75, mostly motor points, listed in the accompanying atlas. Such motor points are the neurovascular hilus points of electromyography where nerve enters muscle. These fewer, physiologically active points were discovered serendipitously in ancient times and later became enshrouded among dozens of lesser or inactive points that, over the centuries, were incorporated into the metaphysical lore of traditional acupuncture.

Studies by Liu (1) and Gunn (2) that compared acupoints with motor points showed a precise concordance with at least 35 points. Many other acupuncture points are located close enough to motor points so that electrical stimulation can activate the motor point even when such a point is not in an exactly concordant position. Gunn (3) described some useful points located at a focal meeting of superficial nerves in the anterior sagittal plane. Other useful points lie over nerve trunks, Golgi tendon organs or nerve plexuses.

Acupuncture meridians are hypothetical and have no demonstrated physiological reality. They are like the longitudinal meridian lines drawn on geographical maps. They may on occasion be descriptively useful as they have for years been a major part of terminology in traditional acupuncture. We have included a list of the commonly used meridian designations for such points (Table III). This list is useful for finding approximate locations for points that one sees in acupuncture literature. The atlas, (Chapter 8), shows the approximate anatomical location of those 75 points that we use and recommend in actual treatment situations.

Tab. III - DESIGNATIONS OF ACUPUNCTURE POINTS USED IN THIS BOOK

LU	Lung
LI	Large Intestine
ST	Stomach
SP	Spleen
HE	Heart
SI	Small Intestine
BL	Bladder
KI	Kidney
PC	Pericardium
TH	Triple heater
GB	Gall bladder
LV	Liver
GV	Governing vessel
CV	Conception vessel
EM	"Extra meridian"

The basic principle of point selection for electrode placement may be simply expressed. It is the location of a body area where electrical stimulation will produce a beneficial change in the central nervous system through modulation of ongoing activity. It is traditional to use only regional points lying within or near neural segments that supply innervation to a given peripheral area of pain. However, recent findings suggest that central action may be more important and that regional placement of electrodes should not be overemphasized. There seems to be a general homeostatic effect regardless of which of the many active points are used. Some points, however, such as the dorsal interosseus motor point of the hand (Figure 24) tend to have larger central cell representation (Figure 25), and hence produce a stronger release of neuropeptides.

b-Trigger points.

At times it may be appropriate to select points for stimulation according to the localization of trigger point reflex pain areas in the manner of techniques elucidated by Travell (4). She described small hypersensitive loci in the myofascial structures that when stimulated, touched or probed, give rise to a larger area of pain in an adjacent or even distant reference area. She noted that such trigger points were more or less constant in their location from one person to another. In our experience they are often in the region of a motor point as shown in the accompanying illustrations adapted from her work, (Figure 26a-d). There is often a concordance of acupuncture points and trigger points. Some of these are the *ah shi* ("ouch") points often used by traditional acupuncturists in the treatment of pain.

Travell postulated that some initial insult sets in motion a chain of events which is thus perpetuated by a continuing cycle of nerve impulses that have no further dependence upon direct afferent stimulation. Rather, they are sustained by a facilitation of the noxious stimulus in closed, self re-exciting chains of internuncial neurons in the central nervous system. The initial stimulus can be a direct trauma to the muscle, chronic muscular strain, chilling, fatigued muscles, acute myositis, arthritis, nerve root injury or visceral ischemia. Peripheral factors include fatigue, chronic infection or psychogenic stress. Electro-acupuncture can act by presumably breaking up such reverberating neuronal circuits.

Protracted myofascial pain following pressure upon trigger points is thought to depend on a reflex pain cycle mediated by the trigger area. Travell reported both temporary and permanent relief from chronic myofascial pain by dry needling of these trigger areas. It is of interest that in some of the trigger/reflex areas she observed that the symptom pattern could be of a complex nature rather than simple pain. Thus, a trigger spot in the sterno-cleido-mastoid muscle, for example, was described as producing dizziness, imbalance, and headaches with at times nausea, vomiting and tinnitus. She also demonstrated the relief of headaches, breast pain, cardiac pain and other symptoms by

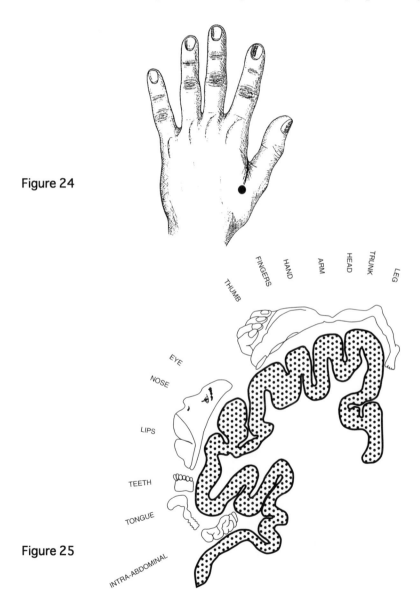

Figure 24

Figure 25

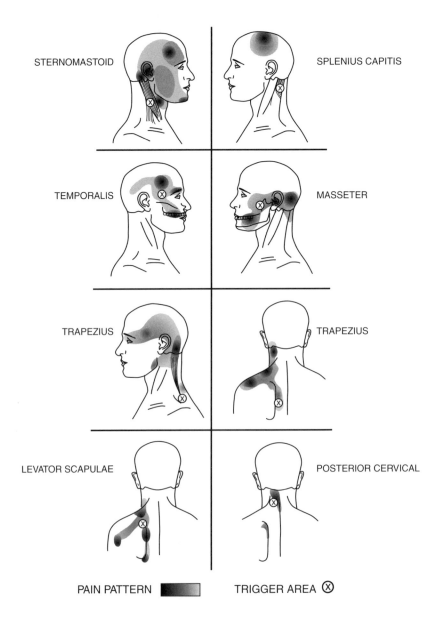

STERNOMASTOID

SPLENIUS CAPITIS

TEMPORALIS

MASSETER

TRAPEZIUS

TRAPEZIUS

LEVATOR SCAPULAE

POSTERIOR CERVICAL

PAIN PATTERN   TRIGGER AREA ⊗

Figure 26a   **Head and Neck**

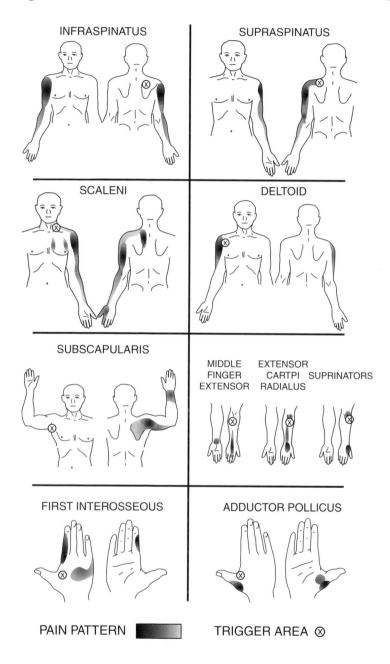

PAIN PATTERN ▮ TRIGGER AREA ⊗

Figure 26b **Shoulder and Arm**

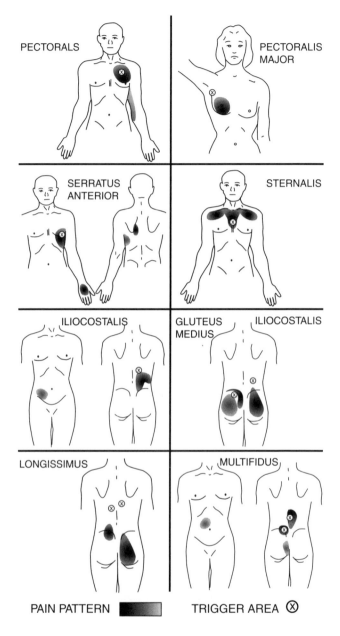

PECTORALS

PECTORALIS MAJOR

SERRATUS ANTERIOR

STERNALIS

ILIOCOSTALIS

GLUTEUS MEDIUS

ILIOCOSTALIS

LONGISSIMUS

MULTIFIDUS

PAIN PATTERN ▮▮▮▮▮   TRIGGER AREA ⊗

Figure 26c   **Chest and Back**

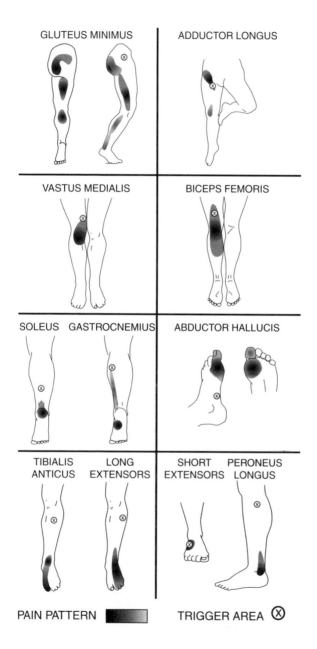

Figure 26d   **Lower Extremity**

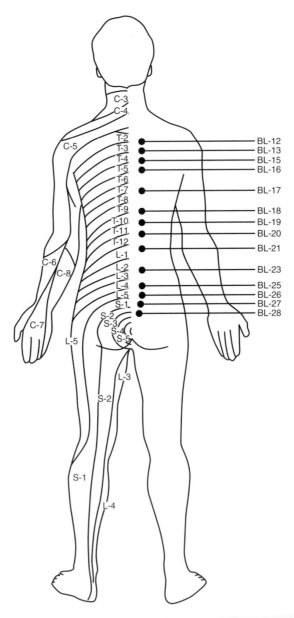

Figure 28   Correspondence of acupuncture meridian "bladder" points
             to spinal neurotome distribution.

stimulation of appropriate cutaneous reference zones for such visceral disturbance.

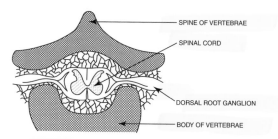

SPINE OF VERTEBRAE

SPINAL CORD

DORSAL ROOT GANGLION

BODY OF VERTEBRAE

Figure 27   **Cross section of vertebral column**

c-Neurotomes

Selection of points for symptom control according to neurotome distribution might be conceptualized according to the gate theory of Melzack and Wall (5). Therapeutic manipulation could be effected either within the troubled neurotome or its corresponding myotome, dermatome or sympathetic ramus. It is necessary to appraise the extent of the discomfort and locate the appropriate spinal segment involved.

Effective points for the treatment of many conditions, therefore, will be found on the dorsal surface of the body on either side of the vertebral column approximately one to two inches lateral to the midline and at the level of each intervertebral foramen at the point where the spinal nerve exits between the vertebra (Figure 27). These correspond to the bladder points of traditional Chinese acupuncture (Figure 28). It is probable that the greatest effect of the stimulation here is through muscle afferents of the posterior rami of the spinal nerves. Depending upon the strength of electrical stimulus, the main nerve trunks (posterior and anterior rami) may be stimulated directly.

Figure 29 illustrates that the palpated vertebral spine does not in all cases correspond to the vertebral body or spinal nerve root of the same number. It will be recalled that as one descends the spinal cord, the nerve roots angle sharply and the nerves must travel longer distances from the shortened spinal cord to the point of their exit from the intervertebral foramina.

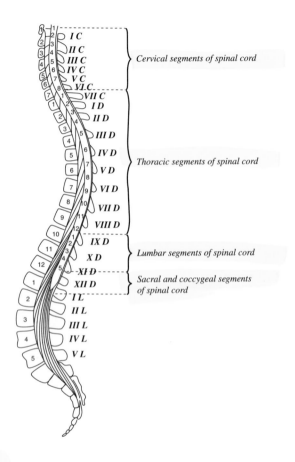

Figure 29

Upon entering the spinal cord, afferent impulses from peripheral nerves may synapse directly for reflex arc function or they may ascend or descend a few segments. Thus it can often be useful to place electrodes above or below the neural level of the lesion either to augment the primary stimulus or, when necessary, to avoid a skin area that may be infected, scarred or otherwise inaccessible to use.

Stimulation of points on the side opposite to the lesion can be effective due to the fact that some fibers cross the spinal cord at or close to the level of the lesion. Such stimulation can be

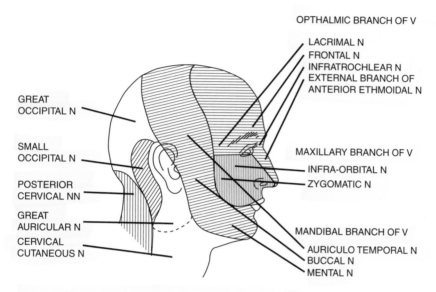

OPTHALMIC BRANCH OF V

LACRIMAL N
FRONTAL N
INFRATROCHLEAR N
EXTERNAL BRANCH OF
ANTERIOR ETHMOIDAL N

GREAT
OCCIPITAL N

SMALL
OCCIPITAL N

POSTERIOR
CERVICAL NN

GREAT
AURICULAR N

CERVICAL
CUTANEOUS N

MAXILLARY BRANCH OF V

INFRA-ORBITAL N
ZYGOMATIC N

MANDIBAL BRANCH OF V

AURICULO TEMPORAL N
BUCCAL N
MENTAL N

Figure 30   **Sensory zones of the head and neck**

blocked by lesions of the cord. In a hemiplegic patient, stimulation of points on the side of the lesion can fail to produce the rise in pain threshold seen following stimulation on the normal side. Similarly, in patients with paraplegia stimulation of leg points can be blocked while points on the upper extremity are still effective.

The importance of segmental neurotome relations has been well demonstrated by Chang of Shanghai (6). He showed that stimulation of the area of the motor point of the sterno-cleido-mastoid muscle produced analgesia sufficient for thyroidectomy. This occurs because cervical nerve C-3 is from the same spinal root that serves the capsule of the thyroid gland. The same principle can apply in treatment of the face. Here areas supplied by sensory innervation are distributed over the three branches of the trigeminal nerve: ophthalmic, maxillary and mandibular (Figure 30). These may also be affected by stimulation of cervical nerve roots because the spinal tract of the trigeminal nucleus reaches downwards to meet ascending impulses from the cervical area (Figure 31).

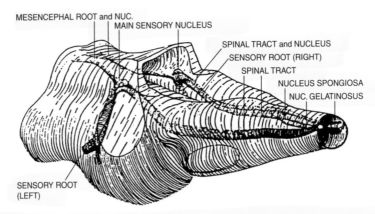

Figure 31   **Location of trigeminal, spinal 5th nucleus in brain stem and
upper cervical cord.** After Kreig, Wendell, J.S.: *Functional Neuroanatomy.* McGraw Hill, New York, Second Edition, 1953

Figure 32 is a diagram illustrating how neurotomes may
overlap. Figure 33a and b, shows diagrams of the neurotome
distribution on the surface of the body together with comparable
illustrations of dermatome distribution. This makes it clear why
an area painful to deep pressure may relate to the spinal segment
innervating the underlying muscle (myotome) rather than the
spinal segment overlying the afflicted spot (dermatome).

It may be appropriate to place the stimulating electrode over
the tender area or motor point of the affected muscle, and as
well, in the paravertebral point of the corresponding neurotome.
Strong stimulation can produce a dull ache, throbbing or draw-

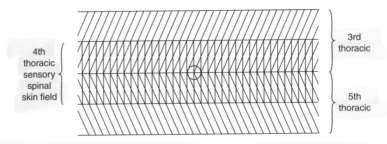

Figure 32   **Scematic illustrating the overlap of dermatomes.** After Ranson,
S.W.: *The Anatomy of the Nervous System.* Sixth Edition. Revised, 1939. Saunders Publishing Company.

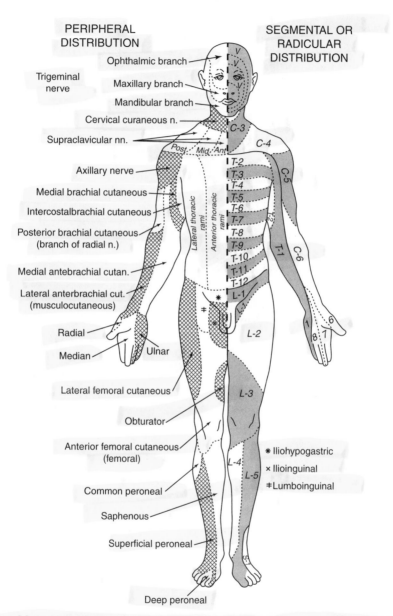

Figure 33a **Neurotome distribution on the human body.** After McDonald, J.J., Green, J.R., and Lange, J.: Correlative Neuroanatomy. Third Edition, 1938. University Medical Publishers, Palo Alto, CA

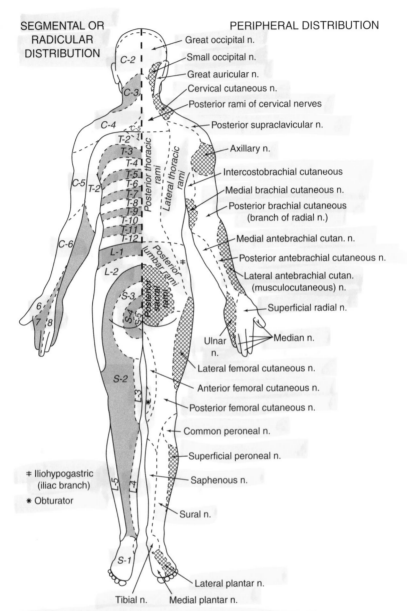

Figure 33b   Neurotome distribution on the human body. After McDonald, J.J., Green, J.R., and Lange, J.: Correlative Neuroanatomy. Third Edition, 1938. University Medical Publishers, Palo Alto, CA

ing sensation such as is seen with deep needle placement. This is referred to in traditional Chinese needle acupuncture as a *Teh Ch'i* or *De Qi* sensation. It occurs when the muscle mechano-receptors are stimulated. At times weak electrical stimulation of dermatome points can produce a counter irritant effect.

d-Cutaneo-Visceral and Viscero-Cutaneous Reflex Points.

Selecting points for the treatment of visceral dysfunction is similar to the selection of points for stimulation within neural segments for referred pain from musculo-fascial structures. Such points of reference have long been known in medicine. Henry Head in 1893 (7) noted the cutaneously referred pain of visceral disease. He demonstrated that counter irritation over the skin and subcutaneous areas of maximal tenderness could alleviate visceral disturbances. He noted that there was often a bilateral distribution of the pain, especially with chronic visceral disturbances. MacKenzie (8) and Kellgran (9) have shown that pain arising from viscera will call into play the cerebrospinal system of sensory nerves with the pain being referred reflexively to the area supplied by the corresponding neurotome. Mann (10) had earlier used the concept of viscero-cutaneous and cutaneo-visceral points to describe the action of some acupuncture points on organs. Weiss and Davis in 1928 (11) noted that referred pain from internally located viscera could be abolished by procaine infiltration of tender areas in the somatic zones of reference, zones that followed patterns often highly consistent from one person to another. Thus, for practical purposes, the segmental distribution of nerves may be of use in selecting effective points for stimulation for the relief of visceral dysfunction.

When disease modifies the function of one organ it can also affect other organs. This is not only because their functions may interrelate, but also because of the spread of neural irritation to adjacent segments up and down the spinal cord. Therefore pain, muscular contractions and vomiting can occur from disturbance of the viscera at any of several locations in the body. The segment of spinal cord stimulated by the afferent autonomic fibers from the disturbed organ can become irritable and produce pain, as well as hyperalgesia of both the skin and the muscles in the external body wall. The area may be remote from the disturbed organ, lie over it or extend widely around it, but in all cases reference to neurotome locations can serve to identify the points for stimulation.

In the living organism there is a succession of stimuli constantly passing from the viscera via afferent nerves to the spinal cord and producing a reflex regulation to maintain homeostasis in muscles, blood vessels, etc. These processes are continually conducted and in such a way that they give rise to no appreciable sensation. If, however, some morbid process occurs in any organ, an imbalance may occur in the homeostatic mechanism. This can affect neighboring nerve cells and can induce a reaction of increased muscle tension in the corresponding myotome or sensory change in the corresponding dermatome. To restore homeostasis it is suggested that the locus of neuro-electric acupuncture stimulation be in the dermatome or myotome that corresponds to the nerve supplying the afflicted organ.

Figure 34 shows the correspondence between certain paravertebrally located acupuncture points and the neurotome segments that innervate body organs. These points (bladder points) are ideally situated for stimulation of the dorsal roots carrying afferent impulses from these organs. Figure 35 illustrates the mechanism of referred pain. In this a stimulus from a dysfunctioning organ (splanchnotome) enters the spinal cord and appears as an area of pain on the body wall (dermatome). Both the organ and the corresponding skin area are served by this same spinal cord segment (neurotome).

On the face, head and neck areas the same principles may be followed. The Chinese have long used the daily massage of points around the orbit of the eye for the promotion of good vision and the treatment of ocular problems. The facial point *Yin Hsiang* (LI-20) has a clinically demonstrated reflex effect upon the mucous linings of the nasal cavity and has thus been useful for the relief of sinus congestion. Translation of the term as "welcome fragrance" speaks directly of its efficacy. Several points around the external ear are believed to have a reflex action, probably vascular, that may produce some relief from eighth cranial nerve afflictions.

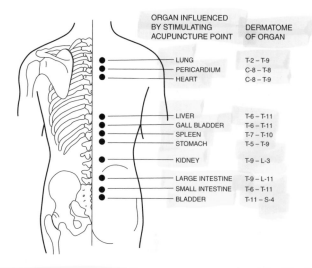

	ORGAN INFLUENCED BY STIMULATING ACUPUNCTURE POINT	DERMATOME OF ORGAN
	LUNG	T-2 – T-9
	PERICARDIUM	C-8 – T-8
	HEART	C-8 – T-9
	LIVER	T-6 – T-11
	GALL BLADDER	T-6 – T-11
	SPLEEN	T-7 – T-10
	STOMACH	T-5 – T-9
	KIDNEY	T-9 – L-3
	LARGE INTESTINE	T-9 – L-11
	SMALL INTESTINE	T-6 – T-11
	BLADDER	T-11 – S-4

Figure 34   **Correspondence between some para-vertebral acupuncture points and neurotome segments that innervate body organs**

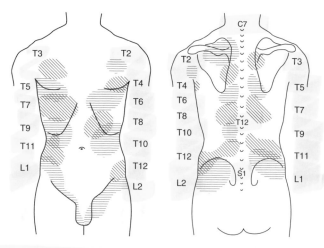

Figure 35   **Distribution of pain on the body wall arising from stimulation of interspinous ligaments. A presumed mechanism for referral of pain from organ dysfunction within the same neurotome.** After Kellgren, J.K.: On the distribution of pain arising from deep somatic structures with charts of segmental pain areas. Clinical Science, 1939-42, 4:35-36

Autonomic effects may be achieved by stimulation not only of the corresponding posterior root but also by reflex action of more distant peripheral points (12). It has been shown by Matsumoto (13) that stimulation of ST-36 can induce peristalsis in post-surgical atony of the gut, both in rabbits and in man. The same point can quiet the increased peristalsis of a colon after the administration of the anti-nociceptive agent CCK-8. Omura (14) has demonstrated that the stimulation of many acupuncture points can produce effects upon micro-circulation. There is initially vasoconstriction followed by a more prolonged vaso-dilitation. It thus appears evident that referred pain and acupuncture share the same pathways of a single neurotome with the skin (dermatome) at one end and the internal organ (splanchnotome) at the other. Thus when disturbance occurs in an organ, pain can be referred to a corresponding skin area. Acupuncture at this point of maximal tenderness can induce a cutaneo-visceral reflex attenuating the referred pain and the visceral disturbance (15).

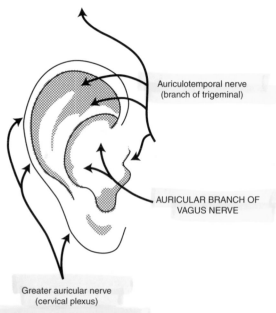

Auriculotemporal nerve
(branch of trigeminal)

AURICULAR BRANCH OF
VAGUS NERVE

Greater auricular nerve
(cervical plexus)

Figure 36   **Innervation of the ear**

Ear acupuncture (auriculotherapy) describes 168 points distributed over the auricle that presumably relate to various parts of the body. It is possible that the effects described arise from a more general central effect from innervation of the ear by branches derived from the trigeminal, facial, glossopharyngeal, vagus, major auricular and the minor occipital nerves. Of these, the vagus is most likely the most important (Figure 36). It is here in the concha that electrical stimulation was first shown to be effective in relieving the autonomic symptoms associated with withdrawal from drugs of addiction (16). The concha of the ear is the only place on the surface of the body where one can easily stimulate fibers of the vagus nerve (Nerve of Arnold). This nerve, a pathway to body viscera, could therefore represent a parasympathetic, homeostatic regulatory mechanism and is well deserving of further scientific research.

e-The treatment

The patient may be in any position in which they will be comfortable for the thirty minute duration of the treatment. This could be in a reclining chair or on a couch or examining table. It is necessary that initially the body area to be stimulated be well exposed. It can then be covered but with care that the lead wires not be entangled. As needles are not used, the patient can shift position slightly as necessary.

Placement of pad electrodes.

Needles are no longer necessary as Han's research has demonstrated that endorphin stimulation occurs equally well with conducting pad electrodes as with electrically stimulated needles at all frequencies tested. Reusable pads may last for 100 or more treatments. For office use disposable pads, such as are used for EKG recording, are preferable (Figure 37). Such pads easily snap onto the stimulation leads. A variety of sizes are obtainable from any medical supply house.

Simply inserting needles into traditional acupuncture points according to ancient formulae is less effective than the stronger stimulation possible with neuro-electrical stimulation of motor points. Increasing the strength of the electrical current will spread the stimulation until the patient's report of *teh chi* indi-

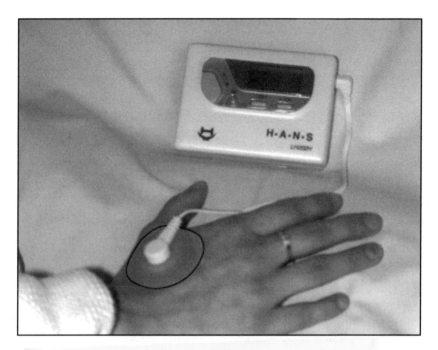

Figure 37   **HANS unit in use for neuro-electric stimulation**

cates that a motor point has been reached. For an optimal effect 30 minutes of stimulation is required. This clearly shows the impracticality of manually twirling needles. As opposed to needles, there have been no untoward complications associated with the use of conducting pads. If needle use is perferred, any radio repair shop can supply leads with small alligator clips for attaching the leads to needles.

There is a saying in ancient China that "the best acupuncturist treats all diseases with but a single needle". Years ago, when I used traditional needle acupuncture, I used many needles with occasional twirling. Now I use an electrical stimulator with two paired leads allowing the placement of four conducting polymer pads on the skin surface (Figure 38). Stimulation of all points can occur simultaneously. With the optimal time of 30 minutes of electrical stimulation, this has served well for most patients.

The aim in all treatments, whether for pain or other conditions, is to assist the body's healing abilities through the restoration of homeostasis. This suggests that the first consideration is stimulation of central mechanisms. Therefore two electrodes are first placed in such fashion as to induce the greatest possible general effect through inducing the gene expression of healing neuropeptides such as endorphins. In order to involve the greatest number of cortical cells for such a general effect we always stimulate the motor point of the dorsal interosseus muscle of the hand. This is the *Hoku*, *Hegu* or LI-4 (Figure 24) point that is the most widely used Chinese acupoint. The second electrode can be placed on the motor point of the adductor policus muscle, directly opposite on the palmer surface of the hand, or else on the wrist or on another nearby point, thus completing the circuit.

The second pair of electrodes is used for stimulation in the area of the patient's complaint. One of the electrode pads can be placed over a trigger point. In China this is often termed an *ah*

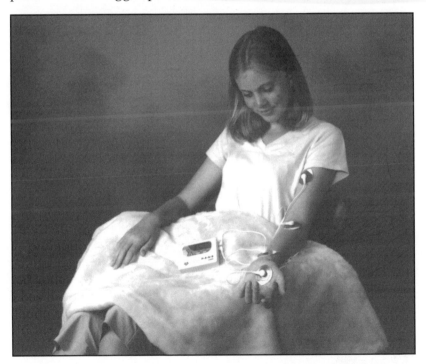

Figure 38   **Multiple pad electrodes stimulated by HANS unit.**

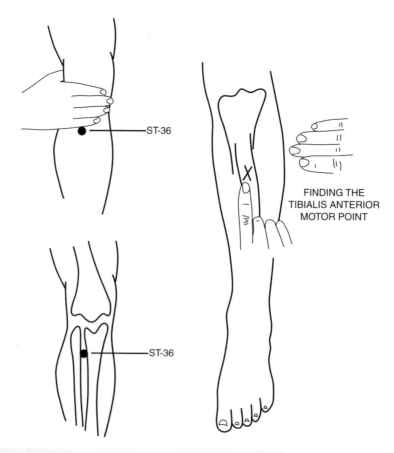

FINDING THE
TIBIALIS ANTERIOR
MOTOR POINT

Figure 39   **Tibialis anterior motor point: ST-36**

shi ("oh yes") point in accord with the patient's response to the physician's probing finger (17). The second electrode of the pair could be placed over the area of the dorsal root of the neurotome innervating the area of discomfort. Such a point would lie within an area not more than two inches from the posterior midline of the vertebral column. These are the bladder points of traditional Chinese acupuncture. If there is no trigger point, the same principle can be followed for any area of general pain or discomfort.

The motor point of the dorsal interosseus muscle of the hand is best suited for stimulation of the upper part of the body through its brachial plexus circuitry. A similar strong point in the lower half of the body is the motor point of the tibialis anticus muscle, *Tsu san li*, or ST-36 (Figure 39). Stimulation here is by way of the lumbo-sacral plexus. This point is found by measuring an approximate four fingers breadth down from the tibial tubercle on the anterior surface of the leg below the patella. The electrode is then placed laterally on the muscle mass lying between the fibula and crest of the tibia. Probing will usually elicit a point of increased tenderness.

The location of motor points and areas of patient's pain from surface landmarks is not an exact matter. With the use of electrical stimulation, however, approximation is sufficient. Electrical current spreads and the intensity of stimulation can be turned up to a point of the patient's maximum comfort tolerance. This assures that the desired bundle of nerve fibers is being stimulated.

Should the patient indicate no specific upper body area of pain, stimulation of the dorsal interosseus muscle areas of both left and right hands may be used. With areas of discomfort in the lower part of the body one of the pair could be on the anterior tibialis motor point with the second electrode placed on an adjacent leg area selected from points shown in the atlas.

The general rule we follow is to:
- First always use one pad on the dorsal interosseus motor point. The second pad can be placed in a nearby area

For the second pair of conducting pads we then consider:
- A trigger point
- A neurotome point for the area of general discomfort
- A motor point

Or
- A point near a major nerve root

Adjusting the stimulation
The preferred stimulation is dense/disperse (D/D) in which a burst of three seconds of 2 Hz stimulation is followed by a burst of three seconds of 100 Hz stimulation. Other frequencies

of stimulation may be used according to the operator's preference, experience or characteristics of the stimulator used.

The intensity of stimulus for each pair of electrodes is adjusted separately. It is not unusual for the patient to feel a difference in sensation between the two electrodes of the pair. When alternating frequencies are used the patient may feel one frequency and not the other. Such differences are not uncommon. It is important that the patient be observed for a minute or two to ensure that the intensity of both pairs of leads is adjusted to a level of comfort. The preferred length of stimulation is thirty minutes.

Frequency of treatment

Treatments are given once or twice weekly until the patient reports considerable relief at which time the interval between treatments may be lengthened. If a patient receives ten treatments with no response it is likely that they are one of the few who are treatment resistant.

Side effects

In our clinical experience with hundreds of patients, no serious side effects have ever occurred. Electrical stimulation of the body in persons with pacemakers should be avoided or performed under supervision by a cardiologist. Although we have experienced no problems, stimulation in the lower half of the body is not recommended in women who are pregnant. Very rarely a patient will report a brief sensation of continuing tingling in the area of stimulation. With careful adjustment of the current intensity, the treatment is a pleasant experience. Most patients feel very relaxed after a treatment and many report an amelioration of pain immediately after and for varying periods of time following a single treatment.

References:

1.   Liu KY, Varela M, Oswald R: The correspondence between some motor points and acupuncture loci. *Am. J. Chin Med* 3:347-358, 1975.

2. Gunn CC: Motor points and motor lines. *Am. J. Acupuncture* 6:55-58, 1978.
3. Gunn CC: Type IV acupuncture points. *Am. J. Acupuncture* 5:51-52, 1977.
4. Travell J: Referred pain from skeletal muscle. *New York State J. Med* 55:331-340, 1955.
5. Melzac R and Wall P: Pain mechanism; a new theory. *Science,* 150:971-973, 1965.
6. Chang, HT: Integrative action of thalamus in the process of acupuncture for analgesia. *Scientia Sinica* 16:25-60, 1973.
7. Head H: On disturbances of sensation with especial reference to the pain of visceral diseases. *Brain* 16:1-133, 1893.
8. MacKenzie J: *Symptoms and Their Interpretation.* London, Shaw and Sons, 1912, p. 304.
9. Kellgren JH: On the distribution of pain arising from deep somatic structures with charts of segmental pain areas. *Clin Sci* 4:35-46, 1939.
10. Mann F: *Scientific Aspects of Acupuncture.* London, William Heinemann Medical Books, Ltd. 1977.
11. Weiss S and Davis D: Significance of afferent impulses from skin in mechanism of visceral pain: skin infiltration as useful therapeutic measure. *Amer J M Sci* 176:517-536, 1928.
12. Chang CY, Chang CT, et al: Peripheral efferent pathways for acupuncture analgesia. *Scientia Sinica* 16:210-217, 1973.
13. Matsumoto T: *Acupuncture for Physicians.* Springfield, IL, CC Thomas, 1974, pp. 204.
14. Omura Y: Patho-physiology of acupuncture treatment: effects of acupuncture on cardio-vascular and nervous systems. *Acupuncture and Electro-Therapy Res.* J. 1:51-140, 1975.
15. Acupuncture Anesthesia Research Group, Morphology Unit, Peking Medical College, Peking Survey of Electric Resistance of Rabbit's Pinna in Experimental Peritonitis and Peptic Ulcer. *Chinese Med J New Series* 2:423-434, 1976.

16. Wen HL and Cheung SYC: Treatment of drug addiction by acupuncture and electrical stimulation. *Asia J Med.* 9:138-141, 1973.
17. Chung C: *Ah-Shih Point, The Pressure Pain Point in Acupuncture.* Taipei, Taiwan, Chen Kwan Book Co., 1982, p. 212.

CHAPTER 8
ATLAS OF USEFUL POINTS

HEAD

Region	Name	Anatomical Location	Physiologic Justification
Vertex	VG-20	Bisection of sagittal line with line joining tragi	Supraorbital n. meets C^2C^3
Temporal	EM-1	At midpoint of a line one fingerbreath to lateral end of eyebrow and outer canthus of eye	Auriculo temporal n. Deep temporal br. of V n.
Supra-Orbital	BL-2	Above supraorbital notch	Corrugator motor point. Supra-orbital br. of V n. Temporal and infraorbital n. of VII n.
Mid-Infra Orbital	ST-1	Just above inferior orbital region	Orbicularis oculi motor point. Infraorbital br. of V n. Facial n.
Median Canthus	BL-1	Just above median canthus	Infratrochlear n. of V
Inferior Masseter	ST-6	Junction of upper 2/3 to lowwer 1/3 of Masseter	Masseter motor point of V

HEAD

Region	Name	Anatomical Location	Physiologic Justification
Anterior Mastoid	TH-17	Posterior to the lobule of the auricle and in the depression between the mastoid process and the ramus of the mandible	Lesser occipital n. C^2C^3 Greater auricular n. C^2C^3
Mandibul-ar	TH-21	With mouth open, temporo-mandibular joint	Auriculo temporal n. Facial n.
Nasolabial Fold	LI-20	Nasolabial fold within the fold of cheek at level of interior edge of ala nasi	Infraorbital br, of V. Buccal br. of VII
Infra-Nasal	GB-26	Midline in the orbicularis oris, 2/3 superior to the margin of upper lip	Infraorbital br. of V Zygomatic br. of VII
Anterior Tragus	SI-19	In front of the tragus at the depression made when the mouth is slightly open	Auriculo temporal br. of V. Facial n.
Lateral Oral Angle	ST-4	1/2 cm lateral to angle of mouth	Orbicularis oris motor point mental n. Cervico facial br. of VII n.

Region	Name	Anatomical Location	Physiologic Justification
Antero-Lateral Mandible	ST-5	Inferior edge of mandible anterior to the gonion, lower anterior border of masseter muscle	Buccal ramus of facial nerve
Anterior Ear	ST-7	Under the zygomatic arch in front of the condyle of the mandible. In the hollow that fills upon opening the jaw	Branches of the temporal and internal pterygold nerves

NECK

Region	Name	Anatomical Location	Physiologic Justification
Sub-occipital	GB-20	Just lateral to trapezius at occiput	Greater occipital C_2 posterior primary ramus
Supraspinous ligament	GV-15	Supraspinous ligament between C_1-C_2 spinous process midline	Posterior ramus C_2 meets C_3
Paracricoid	ST-9	Anterior border of stemomastoid at level of cricoid	Cervical br. of facial n. anteriior cutaneous C_2, C_3
Supra-Sternal	CV-22	Neck extended just above sternal notch	Anterior cutaneous n. of neck C_2, C_3

Region	Name	Anatomical Location	Physiologic Justification
Supra-Spinous Ligament C_7-D_1	GV-14	In the supraspinal ligament, flex head just below C_7 (most prominent spinous process)	Posterior ramus C_3 meets C_4
Stemo-Cleido Mastoid	LI-18	Two fingerbreaths lateral to the mid-point of the laryngeal prominence and between the two heads of the sternocleido-mastoid muscle	Spinal accessory n. (motor) C_2, C_3 (sensory)

UPPER EXTREMITY

Region	Name	Anatomical Location	Physiologic Justification
First Dorsal Space	LI-4	1st dorsal interosseous	1st dorsal interosseous motor point
4th Dorsal Space	TH-3	Between 4-5 metacarpals	4th dorsal interosseous motor point
5th Lateral Metacarpal	SI-3	Ulnar border of and at distal palmar crease (clenched fist)	Abductor digiti quinti motor point

Region	Name	Anatomical Location	Physiologic Justification
Dorsal Distal Forearm	TH-5	3cm proximal to distal end of radius and ulna	Extensor pollicis longus motor point
Dorsal Upper Forearm	TH-9	10cm distal to olecranon	Extensor carpi ulnaris motor point
Lateral Cubital Crease	LI-11	With elbow flexed, at lateral cubital crease	Brachioradialis motor point
Volar Distal Forearm	PC-6	3cm proximal to proximal crease over median nerve	Median nerve
Acromio--Clavicula Joint	LI-16	Acromio-clavicular joint	Supraclavicular n. (C_4)
Posterior Acromion	TH-14	Posterior aspect of acromion	Supraclavicular n. (C_{3-4})
Posterior Axillary Creaase	SI-9	Apex of posterior axillary fold	D_2D_3 meets circulflex n. C_5C_6
Posterior Elbow	TH-10	Posterior surface of arm, just above the point of the elbow, junction of triceps muscle with tendon	Muscle tendon junction Golgi tendon organ

Region	Name	Anatomical Location	Physiologic Justification
Radial Styloid Process	HT-7	Ulnar side of wrist on posterior border of pisiform in depression at radial side of tendon of flexor carpi ulnaris	Medial antebrachial cutaneous n. (T_3); palmar cutaneous branch of the ulnar n. (C_8T_1); Ulnar n. (C_8T_1)
Radial Styloid Process	LU-7	Above styloid process of radius, two fingerbreadths above transverse crease of wrist	Lateral antibrachial cutaneous $(C_{2,8})$. Superficial branch of the radial n.
Top of Shoulder	GB-21	Top of shoulder in midline between C_7 and acromion	Posterior branch of the supraclavicular n. and branches of the cervical plexus
Upper Arm	LI-14	Lateral arm at insertion of deltoid	Auxillary n. posterior cord, posterior division upper trunk C_5C_6

CHEST AND ABDOMEN

Region	Name	Anatomical Location	Physiologic Justification
Anterior Shoulder	SP-20	Second intercostal space 8 fingerbreadths from midline	Motor point of pectoralis

Region	Name	Anatomical Location	Physiologic Justification
Upper Lateral Arm	LU-2	Below the acromial extremity of the clavicle in the depression between deltoid and the pectoralis major	Anterior deltoid motor point
Sub-xiphoid	CV-15	Just below xiphoid process	D_6 and D_7 intercostal anterior cutaneous br. of anterior rami of intercostal
Infra-mammary	ST-18	Over 5th intercostal space at nipple line	Obliquus extremus motor point
Mid-epiga-strium	CV-12	Midpoint between xiphoid and umbilicus	D_8 and D_9 (bilateral)
Lateral Umbilicus	ST-25	Mid rectus abdominus 2 inches lateral to the umbilicus	Rectus abdominus motor point
Upper Hypo-gastrium	CV-6	1/5 distance between umbilicus and pubis in midline	Anterior primary ramus (bilateral) D_{11} and D_{12}
Lower Hypo-gastrium	CV-3	4/5 distance between umbilicus and pubis in midline	Anterior primary ramus (bilateral) D_{12} and L_1 (iliohypogastric)

Region	Name	Anatomical Location	Physiologic Justification
Supra-pubic	CV-2	Just above symphysis pubis	Anterior primary ramus (bilateral) L_1 meets S_2

LOWER EXTREMITY

Region	Name	Anatomical Location	Physiologic Justification
Posterior Trochanter	GB-30	Four fingerbreadths posterior to greater trochanter	Latreal cutaneous nerve of the thigh L_2-L_3
Midgluteal Crease	BL-50	Midline on gluteal fold	Posterior cutaneous nerve of the thigh S_3-S_4
Posterior Mid-Thigh	BL-51	Posterior mid-thigh	Posterior cutaneous nerve of the thigh S_3-S_4
Lateral Mid-Thigh	GB-31	Standing erect, where tip of long finger reaches lateral thigh	Lateral femoral cutaneous N.
Anterior Mid-Thigh	ST-32	5 fingerbreadths superior to the upper margin of patella along the line joining the lateral margin of the patella with the anterior superior iliac spine	Femoral n. posterior division lumbar plexus, L_2, L_3, L_4

Region	Name	Anatomical Location	Physiologic Justification
Medial Supra Patella	SP-10	Three fingerbreadths above upper pole of patella over vastus medialis	Vestus femoral cutaneous n.
Medial Popliteal Crease	BL-54	Middle of popliteal fossa	Posterior femoral cutaneous n. S_2
Lateral Upper Tibialis	ST-36	Four fingerbreadths below lower pole at patella and two fingerbreadths lateral	Tibialis anterior motor point
Anterior Upper Fibula	GB-34	Neck of fibula	Peroneus longus motor point
Mid-Gastro enemius	BL-57	Junction of medial and lateral heads of gastrocnemius in mid-calf at origin of Achilles tendon	Sural n.
Lower Tibia	SP-6	Four fingerbreadths above medial malleolus	Soleus motor point
Posterior Lateral Malleolus	BL-60	Between Achilles tendon and lateral malleosus	Flexor hallicus longus motor point

Region	Name	Anatomical Location	Physiologic Justification
Posterior Median Malleolus	KI-3	Between Achilles tendon and medial malleosus	Superficial branch of saphenous n. L_3-L_4
Second-Third Metatarsal	ST-44	One fingerbreadth proximal to web margin between second and third metatarsals	Superficial peroneal n. (L_5, S_1); Lateral plantar n. ($L_{4,5}$, $S_{1,2,3}$)
Sole of Foot	KI-1	Between second and third metatarsals on sole of foot	Medial plantar n.
Below Medial Malleolus	KI-6	Internal side of leg 2cm below the internal malleosus	Medial branches from the tibial nerve

BACK

Region	Name	Anatomical Location	Physiologic Justification
Para T_2-T_3	BL-12	Erector spinae muscles 3cm from midline para T_2-T_3	Erector spinae motor point
Para T_3-T_4	BL-13	Erector spinae muscles 3cm from midline para T_3-T_4	Erector spinae motor point
Para T_5	BL-15	One fingerbreadth lateral to the inferior end of the spinous process of the 5th thoracic vertebra	Erector spinae motor point

Region	Name	Anatomical Location	Physiologic Justification
Para T_7-T_8	BL-17	Erector spinae muscles 3cm from midline para T_7-T_8	Lower trapezius motor point
Para T_9-T_{10}	BL-18	Erector spinae muscles 3cm from midline para T_9-T_{10}	Lower trapezius motor point
Para T_{10}-T_{11}	BL-19	Erector spinae muscles 3cm from midline para T_{10}-T_{11}	Lower trapezius motor point
Para T_{11}-T_{12}	BL-20	Erector spinae muscles 3cm from midline para T_{11}-T_{12}	Lower trapezius motor point
Para T_{12}-L_1	BL-21	Erector spinae muscles 3cm from midline para T_{12}-L_1	Lower trapezius motor point
Para L_2-L_3	BL-23	Erector spinae muscles 3cm from midline para L_2-L_3	Lower trapezius motor point
Para L_4-L_5	BL-25	Erector spinae muscles 3cm from midline para L_4-L_5	Erector spinae motor point
Para L_5-S_1	BL-26	Erector spinae muscles 3cm from midline para L_5-S_1	Erector spinae motor point
Para S_1-S_2	BL-27	Erector spinae muscles 3cm from midline para S_1-S_2	Erector spinae motor point

Region	Name	Anatomical Location	Physiologic Justification
Para S_2-S_3	BL-28	Erector spinae muscles 3cm from midline para S_2-S_3	Erector spinae motor point
Mid-Back	BL-40	Between sixth and seventh thoracic vertebrae three inches from midline	Trapezius motor point
Sacral Region	BL-49	Level of fourth sacral foramen three inches from midline	Gluteus maximus motor point

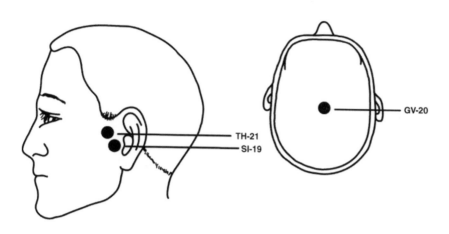

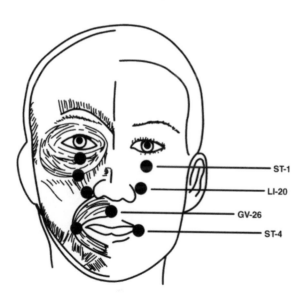

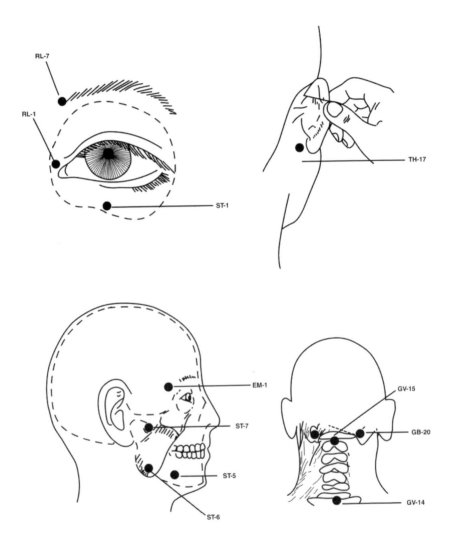

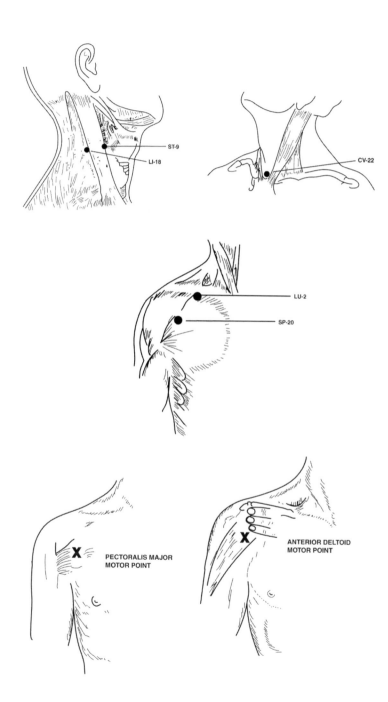

ST-9

LI-18

CV-22

LU-2

SP-20

PECTORALIS MAJOR
MOTOR POINT

ANTERIOR DELTOID
MOTOR POINT

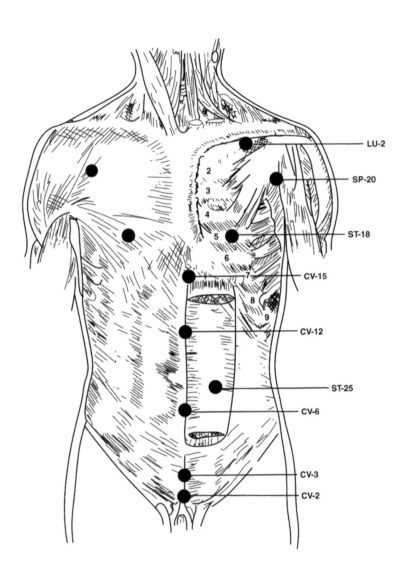

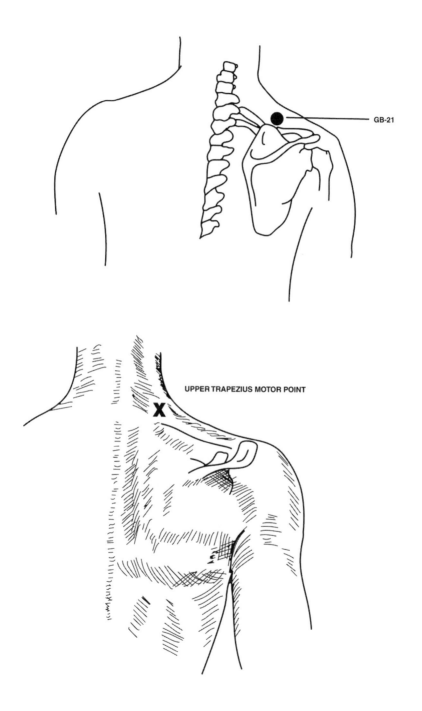

GB-21

UPPER TRAPEZIUS MOTOR POINT

X

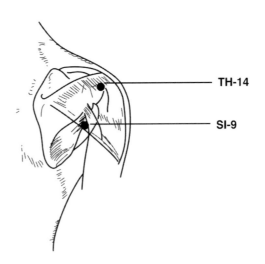

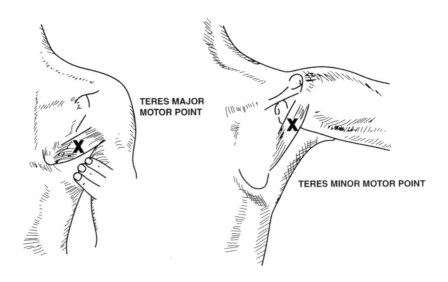

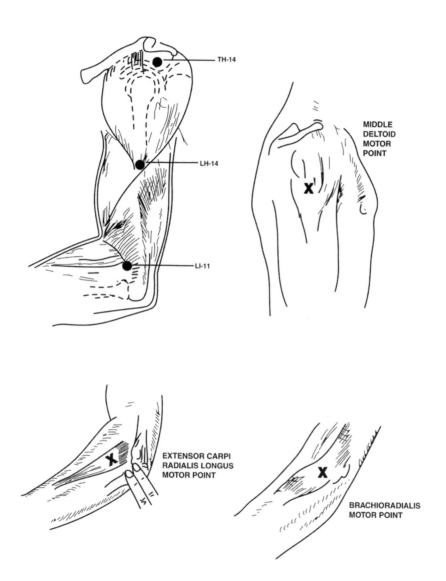

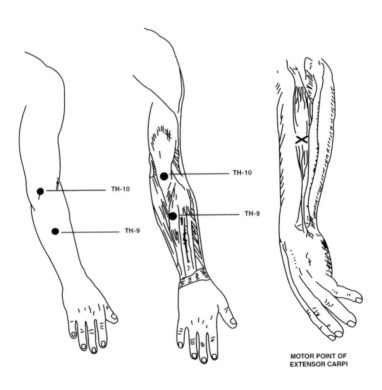

MOTOR POINT OF
EXTENSOR CARPI

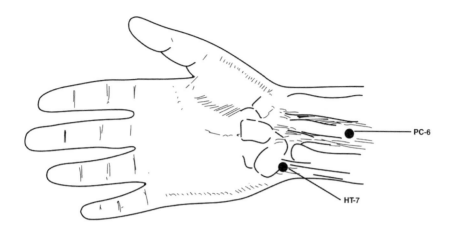

PC-6

HT-7

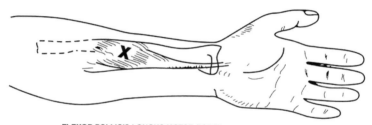

FLEXOR POLLICIS LONGUS MOTOR POINT

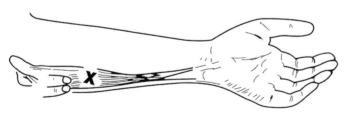

FLEXOR CARPI ULNARIS MOTOR POINT

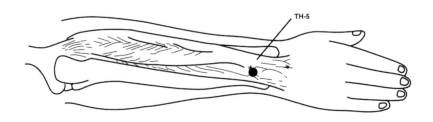

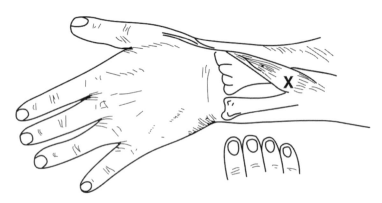

EXTENSOR POLLICIS BREVIS MOTOR POINT

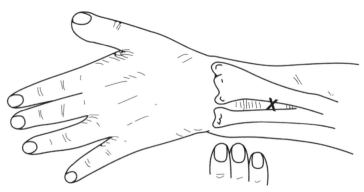

PRONATOR QUADRATUS MOTOR POINT

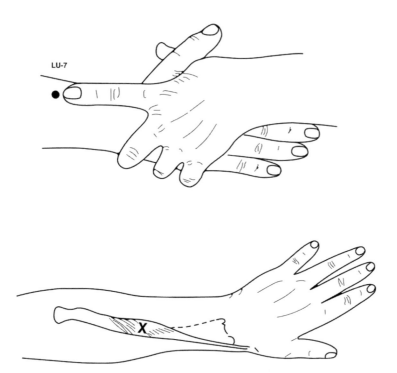

ABDUCTOR POLLICIS LONGUS MOTOR POINT

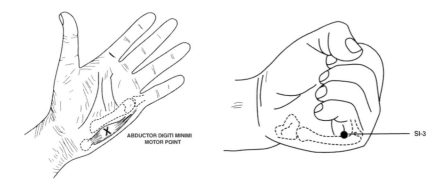

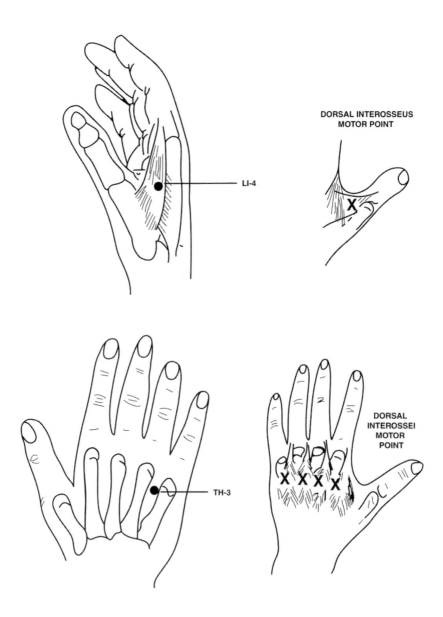

DORSAL INTEROSSEUS
MOTOR POINT

LI-4

DORSAL
INTEROSSEI
MOTOR
POINT

TH-3

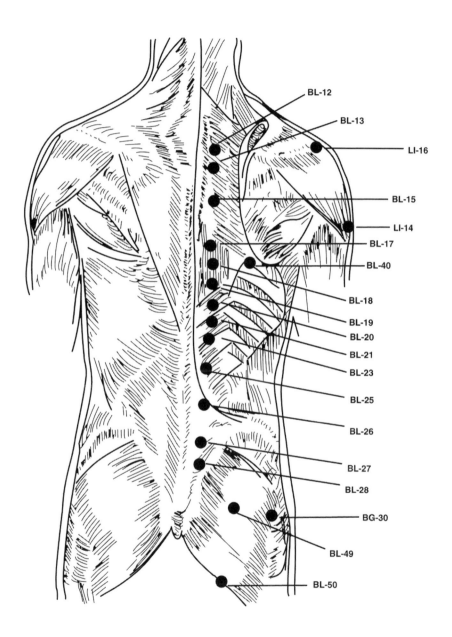

BL-12

BL-13

LI-16

BL-15

LI-14

BL-17

BL-40

BL-18

BL-19

BL-20

BL-21

BL-23

BL-25

BL-26

BL-27

BL-28

BG-30

BL-49

BL-50

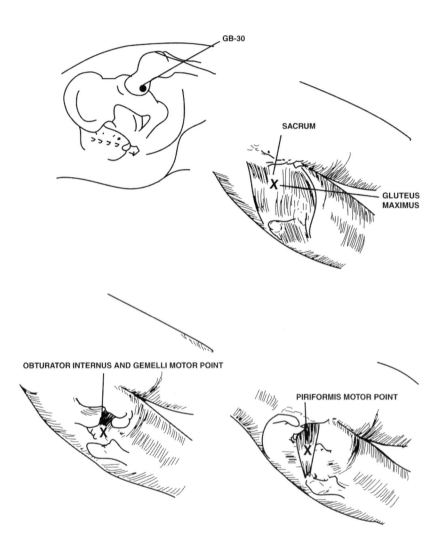

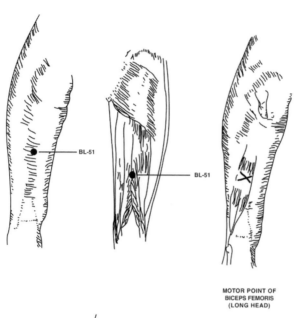

BL-51

BL-51

MOTOR POINT OF
BICEPS FEMORIS
(LONG HEAD)

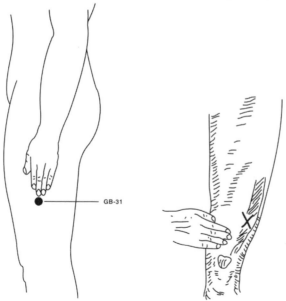

GB-31

MOTOR POINT OF
VASTUS LATERALIS

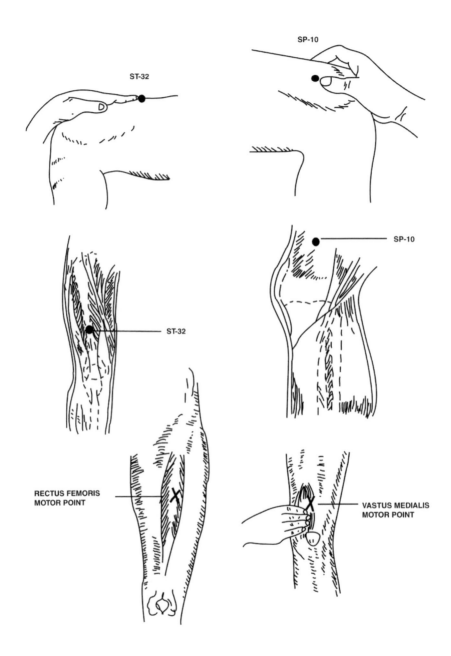

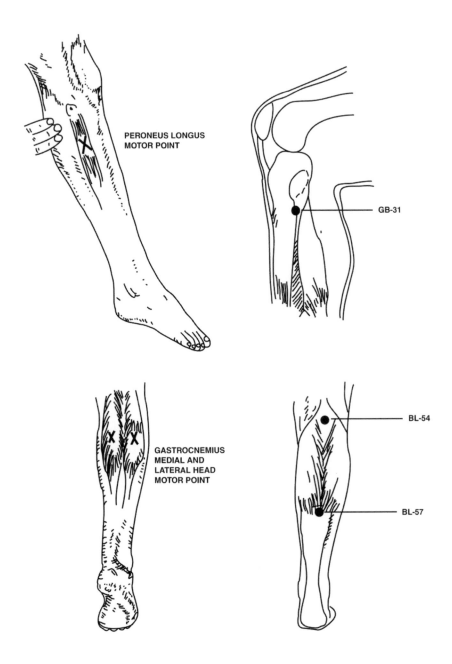

PERONEUS LONGUS
MOTOR POINT

GB-31

GASTROCNEMIUS
MEDIAL AND
LATERAL HEAD
MOTOR POINT

BL-54

BL-57

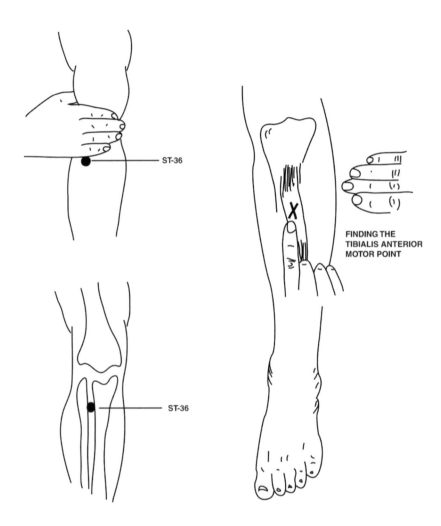

ST-36

ST-36

FINDING THE
TIBIALIS ANTERIOR
MOTOR POINT

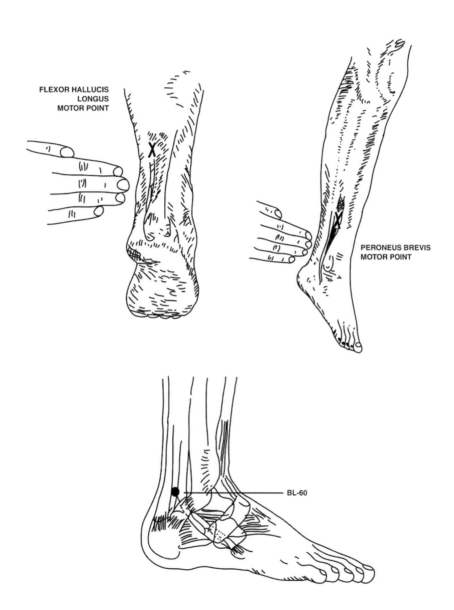

FLEXOR HALLUCIS
LONGUS
MOTOR POINT

PERONEUS BREVIS
MOTOR POINT

BL-60

MOTOR POINTS

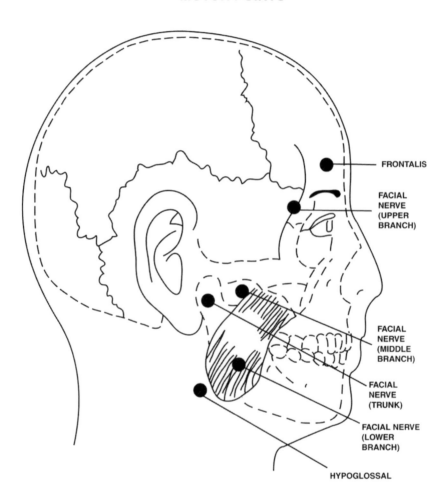

FRONTALIS

FACIAL NERVE (UPPER BRANCH)

FACIAL NERVE (MIDDLE BRANCH)

FACIAL NERVE (TRUNK)

FACIAL NERVE (LOWER BRANCH)

HYPOGLOSSAL

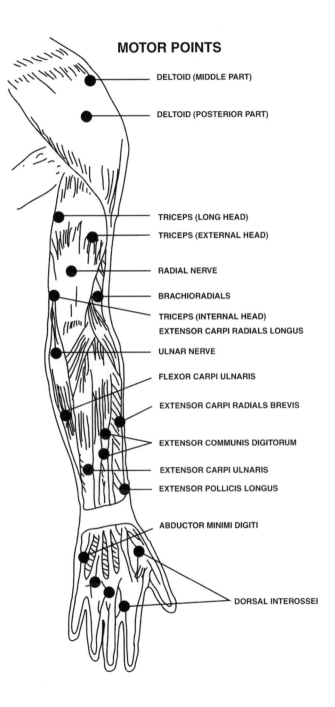

MOTOR POINTS

DELTOID (MIDDLE PART)

DELTOID (POSTERIOR PART)

TRICEPS (LONG HEAD)

TRICEPS (EXTERNAL HEAD)

RADIAL NERVE

BRACHIORADIALS

TRICEPS (INTERNAL HEAD)
EXTENSOR CARPI RADIALS LONGUS

ULNAR NERVE

FLEXOR CARPI ULNARIS

EXTENSOR CARPI RADIALS BREVIS

EXTENSOR COMMUNIS DIGITORUM

EXTENSOR CARPI ULNARIS

EXTENSOR POLLICIS LONGUS

ABDUCTOR MINIMI DIGITI

DORSAL INTEROSSEI

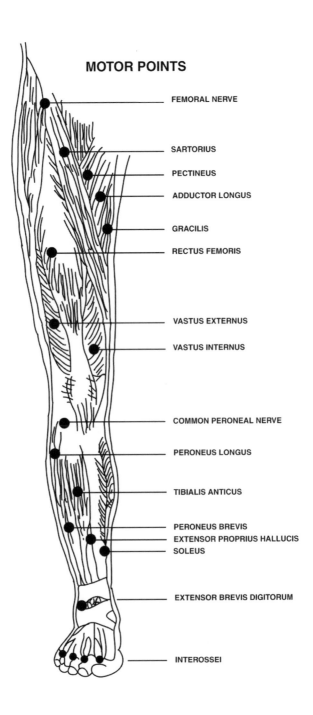

MOTOR POINTS

FEMORAL NERVE

SARTORIUS

PECTINEUS

ADDUCTOR LONGUS

GRACILIS

RECTUS FEMORIS

VASTUS EXTERNUS

VASTUS INTERNUS

COMMON PERONEAL NERVE

PERONEUS LONGUS

TIBIALIS ANTICUS

PERONEUS BREVIS
EXTENSOR PROPRIUS HALLUCIS
SOLEUS

EXTENSOR BREVIS DIGITORUM

INTEROSSEI

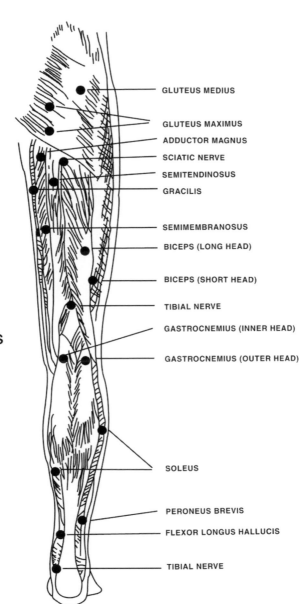

GLUTEUS MEDIUS

GLUTEUS MAXIMUS

ADDUCTOR MAGNUS

SCIATIC NERVE

SEMITENDINOSUS

GRACILIS

SEMIMEMBRANOSUS

BICEPS (LONG HEAD)

BICEPS (SHORT HEAD)

TIBIAL NERVE

GASTROCNEMIUS (INNER HEAD)

GASTROCNEMIUS (OUTER HEAD)

MOTOR POINTS

SOLEUS

PERONEUS BREVIS

FLEXOR LONGUS HALLUCIS

TIBIAL NERVE

CHAPTER 9
USEFUL HINTS AND CASE STUDIES

The number of treatments given depends upon the response of the patient as treatments proceed. Rarely does a patient obtain full relief from a single treatment. Usually during a series of treatments the patient will report gradual improvement. Recording the patient's reports of improvement on a simple linear scale of 1-10 gives an objective way of measuring the effect of treatments. On each visit the patient is asked not "How do you feel today?" but rather "What happened during the week since your last treatment?"

Inquire as to such things as change in degree of pain, change in type of pain, change in location of pain, was there a reduction in amount of medicine taken, improvement in sleep pattern or overall subjective sense of improvement. Approximately 75% of our patients have responded well to a course of treatments. If, after 8-10 treatments, there is no response, the patient may be considered a non-responder.

Treatments are given once or twice a week until the patient is judged to have obtained approximately 50% relief. At this time treatments are given every two weeks. With further improvement, greater spacing between treatments is suggested. Some patients are seen monthly for maintenance of improvement. Other patients will return for booster treatments as needed. In China, patients with serious illnesses may be hospitalized and receive treatments twice a day.

We routinely use electrically conducting polymer pads placed on the surface of the skin for all of our treatments. On very rare occasions, such as when we cannot avoid treatment in a hairy area, we will use an acupuncture needle as an electrode. Disposable stainless steel needles of Chinese or Japanese manufacture are readily obtainable as advertised in journals of acupuncture and alternative medicine. These are very fine, usually 30 gauge, and, due to their extreme flexibility, must be inserted by means of their plastic tube containers. The handle of the needle protrudes from the tube approximately 1/4 inch (Figure 40). Placing the tube firmly against the skin and tapping the protruding end of the handle causes the needle to painlessly penetrate the skin. After the plastic tube is removed the needle can be twisted into the muscle with a drilling motion. This is continued until the patient reports a dull aching or drawing sensation. The Chinese call this sensation *teh chi* or *De Qi,* "drawing of the Qi." It has been demonstrated that this sensation can be blocked by deep intra-muscular procaine but not by subcutaneous injection. This indicates activation of type II and III muscle sensory nerves and can be elicited by electrical stimulation of either conducting pad or needle.

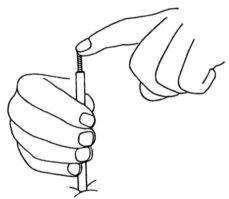

Figure 40   **Inserting a needle**

Simply inserting needles into traditional acupuncture points, according to ancient formulae, is less effective than the stronger stimulation possible with neuro-electrical stimulation of motor points using conducting pads. Increasing the strength of the electrical current will spread the stimulation until the patient's report of *teh chi* indicates that a motor point has been reached. For an optimal effect, 30 minutes of stimulation is required. This clearly shows the impracticality of manually twirling needles. We avoid treating for longer periods of time as this may induce the activation of anti-nociceptive substances such as CCK-8. Contrary to the use of needles, there have been no untoward complications associated with the use of conducting pads.

Illustrative Case Histories

Following are some case histories taken from our files that give an indication of the treatment procedures, electrode placements and clinical results. All of these patients were treated using the HANS stimulator and polymer pad electrodes. The patient's anonymity is maintained by letter designations. Where not otherwise specified, all patients had one pair of electrodes on the "hoku" and on an adjacent point to affect central pain.

J. A. is a 52-year-old male printer who came in with pain in his right shoulder which radiated to the right anterior chest. Patient feels his pain is due to his job which requires much stooping and at times heavy lifting. His physician did a cardiovascular study which was negative and told the patient he thought his pain was primarily due to a muscle condition. Stimulation was, as usual, given to the thumb area on one hand with the two other electrodes placed on shoulder points as shown in the atlas. After six HANS treatments the patient reported much improvement. He felt he would be able to continue working with some changes in his duties.

M. D. is a 55-year-old gentleman who came to my office complaining of migraine headaches. He has suffered from these for many years and had seen many physicians. Medications have not relieved his symptoms. His pain is usually severe and pounding with main location on the left side of his head. One electrode was placed over the point of junction of the tendons of the sterno-cleido-mastoid muscle and upper trapezius muscle where they attach to the occipital bone (GB-20). The other pair of electrodes was placed, as usual, over the LI-4 (*hoku*) point and the opposite palm side of the hand. He was treated weekly for 13 weeks and his symptoms were brought under control. He now receives treatments on a monthly basis.

S. S. is a 37-year-old housewife who complains of lower back pain with pain radiating down her left leg to her knee. Her diagnosis is spinal stenosis with sciatica. One set of electrodes was placed on the ST-36 point of the affected leg with the other electrode on a "bladder" point approximately one inch from the midline at the level of the spinal roots supplying the sciatic nerve. She had ten HANS treatments a week apart and had almost complete relief, but after two weeks she had a return of symptoms. She was given treatments on a monthly basis and these keep her in comparative relief.

J. W. is a 64-year-old widow. She was lifting a suitcase into an airplane overhead rack when the suitcase slipped and she wrenched her shoulder. Now she has chronic shoulder pain. Cortisone injections gave some relief but the pain has returned. Over-the-counter pills upset her stomach. She had HANS treatments in her shoulder area once weekly for three months and the pain has been greatly relieved.

M. G. is a 54-year-old occupational therapist who enters with the complaint of pain in her right heel and back of her leg in an area that has lost sensation. She fell on the ice and suffered a spinal injury at level L4 and L5. There had been but little improvement over the years. She complains of constant pain in the right leg and heel. The usual hand points were the most important. Regional stimulation of the affected neurotome was also given. After seven HANS treatments she made good improvement with lessening of pain.

M. J. is a 70-year-old woman who enters with the chief complaint of pain in her left hip which had been diagnosed as osteoarthritis with radiculitis on the right side. Condition started three years ago with some groin pain. She has had several MRI's which were reported as negative. Treatments were given to LI-4 (*hoku*) as usual and also regionally in the involved neurotome area. After eleven treatments, the patient experienced lessening of pain with increased mobility.

V. K. is a 44-year-old female who enters with the chief complaint of pain in both arms, affecting the fourth digit of both hands. Her condition has been diagnosed as carpal tunnel syndrome. She has tried various therapies but nothing has helped. Electrode pads were placed at elbow and forearm areas in addition to the usual hand points on the affected side. Patient received twelve HANS treatments and stated she had experienced great relief and was now able to continue with her sewing and other hobbies.

J. B. is a 34 year old secretary who had been diagnosed as having a tennis elbow. It began last spring during a tennis match. The pain is in the elbow and spreads toward the hand. One spot on the elbow was sore to touch and evoked the typical pain radiation. This appeared to be a trigger point. One of the electrodes was placed here, the other on a nearby motor point. After 6 treatments the pain began to diminish.

F. E. is a 43 year old widow. She came with pain involving the whole left side of her face. It is a "jabbing" type of pain that comes and goes. She had seen numerous physicians over a five year period but with no relief. One surgeon suggested cutting roots of the trigeminal nerve but told her it would leave her face numb. Electrode pads were placed on various parts of her face, changing their position from one treatment to another. One electrode of the first pair was usually placed over the trunk area of the trigeminal nerve. The other electrode pair was located on the usual hand points. After 12 treatments the pain was gone. It returned a year later. Six treatments were administered and now the pain has been absent for five years.

F. F. is a 47 year old disabled carpenter. Pain is in his right leg which began some years ago with what was diagnosed as "sciatica". He also has diabetes and there is probably vascular involvement contributing to a diabetic neuropathy. He has had several hospitalizations with traction and physical therapy. At times the pain is so severe that he cannot walk. Discoloration, pain and vascular changes led to a diagnosis of "sympathetic reflex dystrophy". A series of ten HANS treatments brought him his "first relief in years". He continues maintenance treatments on a monthly basis.

J. H. is a 49 year old avid fisherman who, every fall, experiences incapacitating headaches. The diagnosis was "cluster headaches". Symptomatic medication helped but did not prevent recurrences. Monthly treatments with the HANS unit served to prevent further headaches.

J. S. has recurrent anxiety attacks and experiences episodes of agoraphobia which are incapacitating. She was given an intensive series of "Conditioning with Electro-acupuncture" treatments. This involved using a 30 minute relaxation tape with music and suggestions for self hypnosis. During neuro-electric stimulation of the LI-4 (*hoku*) pairs of electrodes, bilaterally, she was instructed in relaxing imagery. She was advised to practice the imagery at home for five or ten minutes several times daily. She was also instructed to use this imagery technique whenever she felt the onset of an attack. After a number of weeks of treatments and practice she was able to control her attacks with the conditioned imagery and became relatively free from anxiety.

The above procedure was also used to help persons overcome addiction to cigarette smoking. They were first asked to cut down as much as possible before a set "D-day". On that day they came to the office and destroyed all of their existing cigarettes. They were treated with the conditioning procedure described above twice a week. They carried candy pellets in the usual cigarette case. Thus when the subconscious act of reaching for a smoke occurred they became conscious of what had become an unconscious habit. With this new awareness and armed with the imagery technique for increased endorphin secretion, they were usually able to overcome their habit. The conditioned imagery is then always available should any urge arise. It has helped many break this lethal habit.

The above conditioning/electro-acupuncture technique was used for the out-patient treatment of patients who came with a diagnosis of moderate psychiatric symptoms of depression usually mixed with some anxiety and insomnia. Most were on heavy doses of psychotropic medications and were complaining of uncomfortable and often severe side effects. Almost without exception, we were able to greatly reduce the dependence upon medication and in a number of cases the patients were enabled to stop all medication.

The above cases may serve as examples of our successful treatment techniques. They can be modified to fit the needs of the many kinds of patients who will come seeking help from illnesses that have not responded well to traditional medical care.

CHAPTER 10
PICTORIAL REVIEW OF
ANCIENT METAPHYSICAL ACUPUNCTURE

The question is often asked, "How did Chinese acupuncture originate and why did the Chinese begin to thrust needles into people?" One answer is that body needling was historically a worldwide cultural phenomenon and was not unique to China. Throughout antiquity and in many cultures of the world, even today, body piercing has been practiced as a healing ritual. Trephination, boring into the skull, dates back to early Neolithic times. Instrumental piercing through the intact bony skull was done in order to permit the escape of mystical spirits believed to cause epilepsy and mental illness. In analogous fashion, the body piercing by acupuncturists today is done in accord with ancient ritual, in which the needles penetrate the skin at acupoints on hypothetical meridians in order to free a fancied mysterious *Qi* whose imaginary blockages are the supposed cause of disease.

Nogier, writing on the history of ear acupuncture (auriculotherapy), mentions that 2,000 years ago, in the Mediterranean basin-including Africa, the Mid East, Italy and France, a point on the ear was scarified for the relief of sciatica and other pains. In ancient Egypt a similar point on the skin behind the ear was used as a means of contraception. In the 18th century in Europe, this area was treated by Valsalva to control dental pain.

In China, early skin piercing, "acu" "puncture", was thought to have arisen in prehistoric times accomplished by thorns and bamboo slivers. Excavations of early tombs have uncovered acupuncture needles made of bone. Reports of acupuncture have been found in manuscripts from the middle Chou period (@600 BCE), before the discovery of iron and steel, describing needles made of bronze, copper, gold and silver. Today some acupuncturists ascribe special healing significance to needles fashioned from metals other than steel. Gold needles (yang) are though to stimulate, while silver needles (yin) calm or disperse. Archaeologists have uncovered examples of early needles if various sizes and shapes. Modification of needle shape and size continued as metallurgy improved until today the most commonly used needles are fine steel wires. They come presterilized in plastic tubes to assist with insertion, and they are disposable.

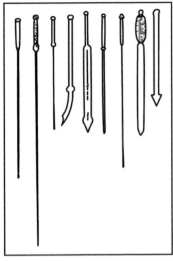

Figure 41   **Ancient needles**

While vision, audition, and olfaction can sample the distant surrounding environment, only the protective organ skin is in intimate contact with our proximate world. Sensors for pain, touch and temperature warn of trouble. These nerve endings in the skin send signals to the brain initiating protective actions as part of the stress response. They can also initiate homeostatic neurochemical cascades leading to healing and comfort. Hence the self reinforcing nature of acupuncture treatments. In addition to methods for penetrating the skin, acupuncturists have devised ways of stimulating the skin's surface by means of corrugated roving wheels and star needle hammers faced

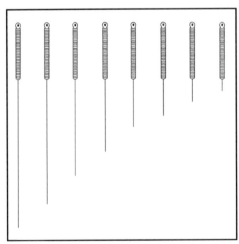

Figure 42   **Modern needles**

with numerous small points. Various methods for chronic stimulation involve the implantation of surgical sutures, tacks held in place by tape and metal surgical staples.

It is probable that special "acu-points" were recognized before there was any systemized acupuncture ritual involving hypothetical meridian channels. Theories and practices differed in various regions of China. Books written in different dynasties showed a gradual pulling together of common threads, but not always with self-consistency. Finally, over centuries, there developed a highly systematized theory of acupuncture practice. It was complex and sophisticated but essentially mysterious as its descriptive underpinning was based largely upon the occult, supernatural beliefs of the ancient 3,500 year old cosmology of the Shang dynasty. No real understanding of these mystical roots of acupuncture can be achieved without reference to the Huang Ti Nei Ching, Su Wen, and Lin Shu *The Yellow Emperor's Manual of Corporeal Medicine*, written probably around the first century BCE. Circulation of the blood was recognized in China before it's discovery by Harvey in the West. This concept added strength to theories of a circulating body energy "Qi" and gave a basis for the complicated system of sphygmology, a diagnostic procedure accomplished by feeling for variations in the radial pulses on the left and right wrists. This is based upon the idea of a supposed representation of twelve organ functions located specifically with six on the yin right wrist, and six on the yang left wrist.

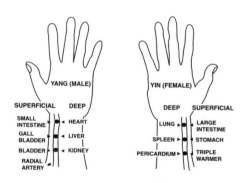

Figure 43   **Pulse diagnosis diagram showing hypothesized locations for detecting supposed changes in energy of body meridians.**

Codifications of acupuncture, as explained in the Yellow Emperor's compendium has remained as the basic conceptual schema to which many elaborations and explanations have been added. Traditional Chinese acupuncture is simply a refinement of these ancient metaphysical beliefs. The previous chapters of this book show that the types of acupuncture in wide use today remain as archaic practices based upon a belief in the mystical concepts of hypothetical meridians and five element theories. These magical rituals have now been made obsolete and superceded by the findings of modern neuro-chemical research.

The following pictures illustrate some points in this discussion and, for historical reasons only, give a pictoral display of figures used in teaching the mystical concepts and rituals of ancient traditional acupuncture.

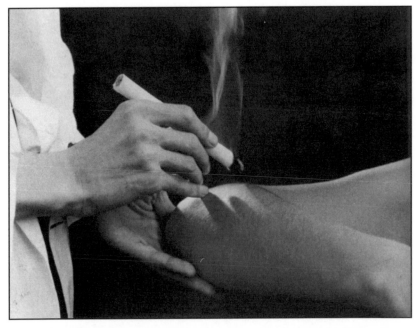

Figure 44   **Moxibustion treatment using a moxa stick (cigar) held over an acupuncture point.**

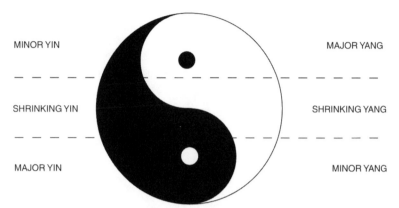

Figure 45   **The waxing and waning of Yin and Yang.**

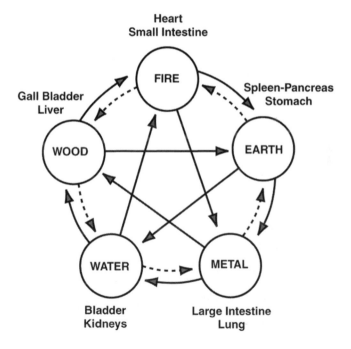

Figure 46   Showing the interaction of the five essences and how they may influence one another. Clockwise rotation is the engendering (strengthening) sheng cycle. Counterclockwise is the overcoming (weakening) ko cycle.

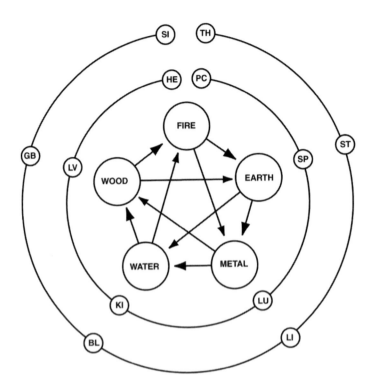

DOCTRINE OF THE FIVE ELEMENTS "THE LAW OF WU HING"
Illustrating How These Elements Exercise an
Influence Upon One Another

THE SHENG CYCLE	THE KO CYCLE
FIRE engenders EARTH	FIRE overcomes METAL by melting
EARTH engenders METAL	METAL overcomes WOOD by cutting
METAL engenders WATER	WOOD overcomes EARTH by covering
WATER engenders WOOD	EARTH overcomes WATER by damming
WOOD engenders FIRE	WATER overcomes FIRE by extinguishing

Figure 47   The changes in Figure 47 (as opposed to the diagram in Figure 46) were adopted to adjust five element theory to meridian theory with pulse diagnosis requiring the symmetry of six pulses on each wrist, hence, the fire element is split to accomodate two additional meridians, the TH (triple heaters) and PC (pericardium).

The following three figures are maps of the body and organs located in the ear (auriculotherapy), foot (reflexology) and hand (Korean acupuncture). That such points appear specific for the body regions indicated lacks scientific anatomical confirmation. The apparent specificity from needle stimulation nay be explained in terms of fMRI crossmodal spatial attention studies which show that an entering sensory stimulus can have widespread connections in the brain.

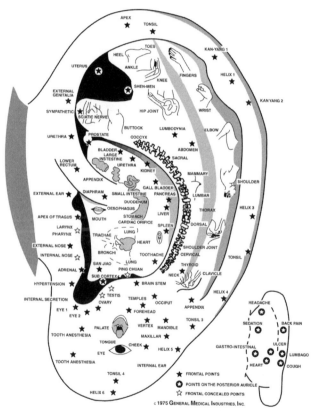

Figure 48   Correspondence between designated points on the auricle and regions of body anatomy as theorized by auriculotherapists. Note that the major body organs, which are innervated by the autonomic nervous system, lie within the concha of the ear, an area supplied by the vagus nerve.

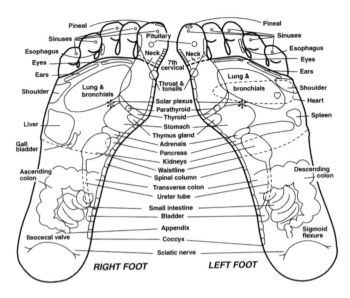

Figure 49   **Reflexology map**

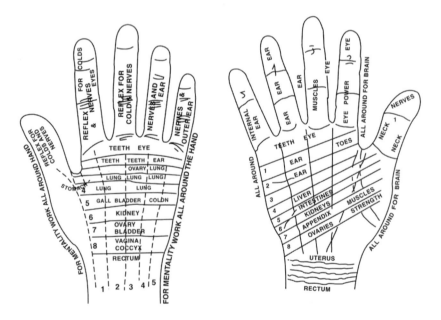

Figure 50   **Korean acupuncture map**

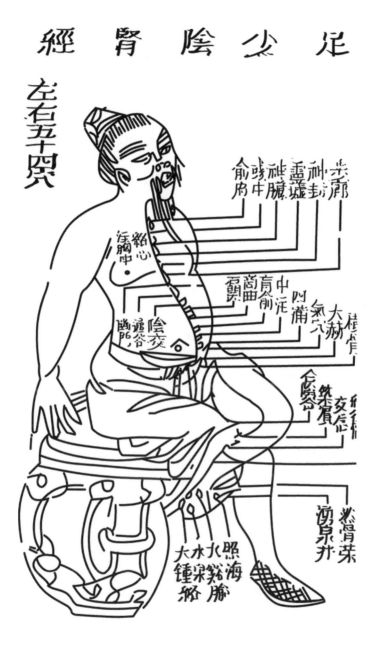

Figure 51 **An early chart of a meridian shown with acupoints.**

References:

1. Gwei-Djen, Lu and Needham, J. *Celestial Lancets: A History and Rationale of Acupuncture and Moxa.* Cambridge University Press, Cambridge, 1980.
2. Ulett, G. *Beyond Yin and Yang: How Acupuncture Really Works.* Warren Green Publishers, St. Louis, 1992.
3. Nogier, P.F.M. *Treatise of Auriculotherapy.* Maissonneuve, France, 1972.